“Divulging of Useful Truths in Physick”

"Divulging of Useful Truths in Physick"

The Medical Agenda of Robert Boyle

BARBARA BEIGUN KAPLAN

The Johns Hopkins University Press
Baltimore and London

Printed in the United States of American on acid-free paper

The Johns Hopkins University Press
2715 North Charles Street
Baltimore, Maryland 21218-4319
The Johns Hopkins Press Ltd., London

Library of Congress Cataloging-in-Publication Data

Kaplan, Barbara Beigun, 1943–
"Divulging of useful truths in physick" : the medical agenda of Robert Boyle / Barbara Beigun Kaplan.
p. cm.
Includes bibliographical references and index.
ISBN 0-8018-4601-3 (hc : alk. paper)
1. Boyle, Robert, 1627–1691. 2. Medicine—Great Britain—History—17th century. I. Title.
[DNLM: 1. Boyle, Robert, 1627–1691. 2. History of Medicine, 17th Cent.—England. 3. Philosophy, Medical—England. WZ 70 FE5 K17d 1993]
R489.B693K37 1993
610'.92—dc20
DNLM/DLC
for Library of Congress 92-48468

A catalog record for this book is available from the British Library.

To my parents

Jack L. Beigun

Mollie Schulman Beigun

And therefore I reckon the investigation and divulging of useful truths in physick . . . among the greatest and most extensive acts of charity . . . by which a man may . . . oblige mankind.

Robert Boyle
The Usefulness of Natural Philosophy

TABLE OF CONTENTS

PREFACE

Robert Boyle holds a special place in the history of science as a well-lettered seventeenth-century English virtuoso and experimenter. Boyle's contributions to the history of chemistry and his researches into pneumatics have been well documented, and his espousal and popularization of a corpuscular theory of matter as a groundwork for his views has also been emphasized. Because of his wide-ranging interests, however, Boyle is a significant figure in areas other than chemistry and physics. His theological works reveal that he was a deeply religious thinker who, like many others in his century, sought the reconciliation of science and Scripture for the greater glory of God. His meditative notes show him to be a contemplative humanist. His medical writings—the subject of this study—present Boyle as actively engaged in research relevant to medicine and directly involved with some of the most fundamental questions of his day regarding the physician's proper approach to his discipline.

Because Boyle was held in high esteem by his contemporaries, his opinions were frequently requested and highly valued. Despite his lack of formal medical training, Boyle's familiarity with medicine was broad, and his suggestions for improvements within that science were extensive. His specific ideas of medicine thus become important to an assessment of the history of English medicine in the mid-seventeenth and early eighteenth centuries. It is my purpose here to describe and analyze Boyle's medical ideas in order to determine the scope and the degree of sophistication of his medical thought.

My research was greatly facilitated by the kind assistance of the people connected with the National Library of Medicine in Bethesda, Maryland, and the staff of the Library of the Royal Society in London. Particular acknowledgment is due to Dr. John Duffy and the late Dr. Francis Haber, my professors and mentors, for their guidance and inspiration. I am greatly indebted to Jacqueline Wehmueller, of the Johns Hopkins University Press, for her many kindnesses and her unflagging support for this project. To my children, Jeff, Eric, Brian, and Robyn, who endured many inconveniences while I was preoccupied with writing at home and yet gave constant encouragement to my efforts, and to my husband Howard, who willingly served as a sounding board for my many random thoughts, I convey my deepest thanks for their indispensable moral support. Finally, to my mother Mollie Schulman Beigun, whose unfailing faith in me has always provided a much-needed prop in difficult times, I owe a gratitude beyond measure.

"Divulging of Useful Truths in Physick"

Introduction

A conspicuous feature of mid-seventeenth-century English medical thought was its diversity. Attacks on traditional Galenic doctrine and the methodological confusion caused by attempts to incorporate new empirical information and new theoretical perspectives into the professional practice of medicine frequently resulted in bitter debates over the proper rational basis for the physician's diagnostic and therapeutic decisions.

These debates, which first challenged and eventually reshaped the *methodus medendi* of the Galenists,[1] were part of the intense scrutiny of traditional Scholastic thought that had begun in the Renaissance. The substance of these debates was of considerable interest to people outside the medical community. The political, religious, and intellectual turmoil of mid-seventeenth-century England amplified and hastened this reappraisal of traditionally held knowledge and also prompted a particularly keen interest in social welfare and the improvement of the human condition. Medicine became a public subject in this age, and medical reform was urged in many quarters. It is not surprising, therefore, to discover that many intellectuals who were not themselves physicians chose to write and converse extensively about the proper method of medical investigation and the nature of the physician's role in curing disease.

One such man, whose writings reveal an intense personal interest both in the medical thought of his day and in broader questions of scientific methodology and medical reform, was the self-styled "natural philosopher" Robert Boyle. Best known to us for his contributions to chemistry and pneumatics, Boyle was an important popularizer of science as well as the patron of many who espoused the new mechanical philosophy. Boyle's articulation of the "corpuscular hypothesis" and his specific suggestions for an empirical methodology in science should be appreciated as a sophisticated attempt to create a logically consistent foundation for understanding the operations of nature. Medicine for Boyle was an important subset of natural philosophy. He effectively argued that organized investigation by open-minded, cooperating researchers held the best hope for improving knowledge of physiology and disease and that this knowledge would provide the means to achieve meaningful medical reform. Boyle's religious convictions, and especially his attachment to irenical Protestantism, also contributed significantly to the development of his ideas on collaborative medical investigation.

Religious sectarianism was rife in Boyle's day, and so was medical factionalism. Often, in fact, the radical sectaries were among the most vocal advocates of medical reform. Opposed to divisiveness and committed to a social order in which change would come about through reason and consensus, Boyle promoted a broad-based empirical method, which he hoped would unite disparate parties and result not only in practical benefits for science in general but also in improvements in human health. The repeated references Boyle makes to medicine in his writings should not be dismissed as the casual dabbling of an eclectic scientist; rather, they should be seen as reflecting a sincere desire to integrate medicine into his larger vision of scientific advancement.

Boyle, who was thoroughly acquainted with both traditional and contemporary medical literature, numbered among his friends medical practitioners who espoused a wide variety of theories. In his writings he reveals a familiarity with almost every major medical discovery or theory occupying the attention of physicians of his day. Although he often used examples from medicine to highlight the potential practical value of his corpuscular philosophy, his references to medicine were far more than illustrations for his philosophical arguments. His extensive discussions of the causes of disease (particularly airborne epidemic diseases), of physiological function, of the importance of anatomy studies and dissections to medical studies, of the proper role of the physician, and of the use and preparation of drugs have, overall, a logical consistency and a high degree of sophistication. In the course of his own laboratory research, Boyle also made some specific contributions, which, although not major discoveries, proved useful to medicine and pharmacy.

Boyle's significance to the history of medicine should be appreciated, therefore, on several levels. As a researcher, Boyle sought to discover specific facts that could directly benefit the physician. As a Christian philosopher, he tried to provide a conceptual foundation for understanding human physiology and disease that also took into account God's divine plan of creation. As a moralist concerned with Protestant unity and promotion of the common good, he aimed at encouraging individuals to be responsible for promoting the general welfare and to pool their exper-

"Divulging of Useful Truths in Physick"

tise so that the quality of life could be improved. As an advocate of the new science, he promoted the idea that rational explanations of the operations of nature were possible using his corpuscular views of matter and that there was no need to posit occult forces or directive "faculties" even in discussions of complex life processes.

Boyle's views on medicine have received some attention from modern scholars, but there has not been a detailed account of his medical ideas and their place in the medical thought of his time. To Boyle's own contemporaries, however, his strong medical interests were very apparent. He was often consulted for medical advice, and he shared recipes and remedies with his friends. Boyle is known to have suggested medical topics for his colleagues to investigate. His friend Thomas Sydenham, a physician, permitted Boyle to accompany him in attending patients. There is evidence that Boyle received the degree of "doctor of physick" from Oxford in 1665, and although this was probably conferred as an honorific, the fact that it was the only degree he ever received should indicate something of the esteem in which his medical efforts were held.

The modern scholar seeking to understand the scope and structure of Boyle's medical thought must, of necessity, undertake the task of comprehending the totality of Boyle's extensive and prolix writings. Crucial to our understanding of Boyle's philosophy is the fact, already mentioned, that Boyle considered medicine a subcategory of natural philosophy and therefore subject to the same methods of fact-gathering and data verification as other natural phenomena. His comments on topics pertinent to medicine were usually incorporated into treatises dealing with the larger subject of the proper study of nature. As a result, although there are some important works in the Boyle corpus specifically devoted to medicine, we find references to his methodological and theoretical views concerning medicine in a variety of treatises. It is also true that Boyle's method of work was disorganized, and he often lifted passages from a draft of one work to place in another. It is necessary, therefore, to consider his literary production in its entirety in order to interpret and evaluate adequately the whole of his medical viewpoint.

A salient characteristic of Boyle's thought, and one that, as we shall see, distinguished his medical views from those of stricter mechanists such as Descartes, was his insistence that the human body could not be understood in isolation from the whole of creation. The greater world of nature and the smaller world of the human body formed an interrelated whole, and to study the human body as a separate, isolated system was inappropriate. (This is another reason why he so often chose to discuss medical ideas in treatises dealing more broadly with the study of nature.)

Physicians could improve their craft most, Boyle thought, by viewing human physiology and the conditions relating to health and disease within a holistic context.

Boyle insisted that any learned individual could further the progress of medicine by providing insights that the trained physician could use to improve his understanding of the functioning of the human body. This collective approach to knowledge, popularized by the writings of Francis Bacon, became an intrinsic part of Boyle's general scientific methodology. Boyle's idea that any reasonable observation about the human body or about a potentially effective cure (even those forwarded by nonphysicians) should be seriously considered by the professional medical community was articulated clearly in his *Experimenta et Observationes Physicae* (1691), where he stated: "Natural philosophy being a science of far greater extent than physic, and supplying it with many of its principles and theories, it is very possible, that naturalists, though not professed physicians, may propose some such comprehensive notions and methods, as may awaken and enlarge the minds of them that are so, and at least afford some useful hints to considering and ingenious men."[2] Boyle firmly believed that physicians must abandon their traditional reliance on authority and adopt an open-minded approach in order to improve their craft. This emphasis on proper attitude was, in fact, a key element of his medical perspective. Yet he recognized that he could only persuade physicians to accept the value of this approach by gentle encouragement supported by reasonable argument. The nondogmatic and cautious way Boyle presented his arguments was, as we shall see, both a help and a hindrance to the acceptance of his views by the professional medical community.

Before focusing on the specifics of Boyle's medical thought, it may be useful to identify which of his many works contain significant medical subject matter. The following summary indicates the scope of his efforts and lends credence to the notion that Boyle's interest in medicine was lifelong and pervasive. The treatise of Boyle's that contains the most organized store of medical information is unquestionably his *Usefulness of Experimental Natural Philosophy.* Part 1 of this work was written quite early, around 1650, and reflects a major theme in Boyle's writings, namely, that experimental science is a laudable endeavor for man because it familiarizes him with God's creation and leads to useful discoveries that contribute to human welfare. Part 2, written about 1658, deals specifically with medicine as an example of a useful art that can be augmented by the experimental investigator. Boyle meticulously outlines the value of experimental inquiry to the five traditional categories of medical knowledge—physiological, pathological, semeiotical (dealing with signs or symptoms of disease), hygienal, and therapeutical. He maintains that no adequate understanding of the human body and its functions is possible without a basic knowledge of anatomy, physics, and chemistry. Although Boyle cautions that one never can hope to gain certainty about the physical operations of so complex a creation as the human body, he insists that the skilled natural philosopher can supply information to aid the physician in perfecting his craft.

Boyle published this treatise in 1663. A second edition appeared in 1664. Boyle's publication of this work at this particular time was motivated at least partly by his desire to justify the scientific activities of the newly created Royal Society of London, the organization to which he devoted so much of his own energy. In arguing for the usefulness of broad-based knowledge, Boyle reveals many of his own thoughts on drug action, disease causation, and physiological function.

Another key area of Boyle's investigations was respiration. As is well known, Boyle devoted many treatises to the general subject of the air. In these one finds not only his detailed experiments attempting to link respiration and combustion but also important speculative passages dealing with the role of the air in the production and transmission of disease. Boyle's first signed published work, *New Experiments, Physico-Mechanical, Touching the Spring of the Air* (1660), focused on the subject of respiration. In a follow-up work, "New Pneumatical Experiments about Respiration," published in *Philosophical Transactions,* 8 August 1670, he detailed his experiments upon animals in his vacuum receiver. In 1672 he explored the possibility of a connection between respiration and combustion in *New Experiments about the Relation between Air and the Flamma Vitalis of Animals.*

Meanwhile, in 1671 Boyle appended to his *Tracts about the Cosmical Qualities of Things* a section entitled *Cosmical Suspicions* in which he speculated that periodic changes in the atmosphere can cause anomalies in nature, including the creation of specific diseases. He continued to question possible effects of the air upon the human body in other works published during the 1670s and 1680s. In the *Philosophical Transactions of the Royal Society,* 24 February 1672/73,[3] Boyle published "A New Experiment concerning an Effect of the Varying Weight of the Atmosphere upon some Bodies in the Water; suggesting a Conjecture, that the very Alterations of the Air, in point of Weight, may have Considerable Operations, even upon Men's Sickness or Health," in which he speculated that changes in atmospheric pressure might affect air particles contained within the pores of the blood, causing an interference with circulation, which could lead to illness.

In 1673, in *Essays of the strange Subtilty, great Efficacy, determinate Nature of Effluviums,* Boyle discussed more fully ideas he had first presented in *Cosmical Suspicions* regarding the effect that particles emitted from various bodies into the air can have upon other bodies with which they come into contact. The year 1674 saw the publication of Boyle's *Suspicions about some Hidden Qualities of the Air,* in which he put forward the view that a "vital substance" present in the air is necessary for the sustenance of flame. He also discussed the possibility that the heterogeneous effluvial particles carried by the air might interact chemically with each other, causing changes in the temperature and constitution of the atmosphere, which could thus give rise to pestilential diseases. Boyle continued his exploration of effluvial activity in 1685, in an appendix to his *Essay of the Great Effects of Languid and Unheeded Local Motion* entitled "Experimental Discourse of Unheeded Causes of the Insalubrity and Salubrity of the Air." Here Boyle suggested that effluvial particles transmitted through the air insinuated themselves into the human body either through the pores of the skin or via respiration and disrupted body processes by promoting inordinate motions and chemical alterations.

Another group of treatises by Boyle was devoted specifically to the subject of medicinal remedies. Henry Oldenburg's Commonplace Book for 1660 contains a fragment of a very early work by Boyle, "An Essay of Turning Poisons into Medicine," which deals with methods of altering various poisonous substances for medicinal use, a notion common in Paracelsian medicine.[4] Boyle quotes a small passage from this treatise in his *Usefulness of Experimental Natural Philosophy,* noting there that he has chosen "for certain reasons" (probably ethical) to suppress the work as a whole.[5] In the section of *Certain Physiological Essays* (1661) entitled "Of the Unsuccessfulness of Experiments," Boyle considered variables that could prevent a given remedy from working properly. He noted that medicine was a field especially subject to failed experiments for which no accountable explanation could be ascertained.

In 1672 Boyle took up the question of the medical efficacy of gemstones. In *Origin and Virtues of Gems* he rejects the traditional occult interpretation of the curative power of gemstones in favor of corpuscular and chemical explanations.

Boyle's most important work on the subject of drug action was *Of the Reconcileableness of Specific Medicines to the Corpuscular Philosophy,* published in 1685. Convinced that specifics had an important future in medical therapeutics, he sought to explain their efficacy on the basis of corpuscular interaction. In an appendix entitled "The Advantages and Uses of Simple Medicines," Boyle argued that remedies composed of only one or two ingredients were preferable to more complex remedies, not only from the perspective of the patient, who would experience fewer side effects, but also from the view of the physician seeking verification of the effects of particular drug substances upon the individual.

In 1688 Boyle published a collection of medicinal remedies entitled *Receipts sent to a Friend in America.* (This collection was expanded to include additional recipes in a posthumous second edition in 1692 entitled *Medicinal Experiments, or a Collection of Choice and Safe Remedies, for the most Part Simple, and Easily Prepared: Very Useful in Families, and fitted for the Service of Country People.*) This work exemplifies the genre of medical recipe books, popular in the mid-seventeenth century, that were written in the vernacular and designed as self-help manuals. In Boyle's case, this work also reflects his religious commitment to improve the human condition (such activity being required of the pious Christian gentleman) and is consistent with the therapeutics-based medical reform he espoused. The actual collection of recipes in this work is rather haphazard, although Boyle makes some attempt to rate the efficacy of various prescriptions. In a third edition, in 1698, a third volume was added; however, John Fulton considered this third volume to be spurious.[6]

In the last work published during his lifetime, *Experimenta et Observationes Physicae* (1691), Boyle also included information on chemical remedies and provided some interesting medical case histories. Essentially a collection of experiments on various subjects, this work reveals that even to the end of his life Boyle was anxious to impart even random suggestions and recipes in the hope that these might prove useful to medicine. Here again he asserts his conviction that the trained chemist can provide significant insights into the medical art.

Two additional treatises by Boyle show how valuable chemical knowledge could be for medicine. His *Short Memoirs for the Natural Experimental History of Mineral Waters* (1684/85) suggests ways of determining the specific chemical content of mineral springs (primarily by use of color tests) to enable physicians to determine their particular medical usefulness. Boyle's *Medicina Hydrostatica,* published in 1690, details the method of determining relative specific gravities for the purpose of judging the purity of drug substances. Despite its brevity, this latter work should be considered one of Boyle's most innovative and a major contribution to pharmacology.

Typical of some other medical investigators of his time, Boyle became interested in the implications of Harvey's discovery of the circulation of the blood. In *Memoirs for the Natural History of the Humane Blood* (1683), Boyle detailed his suggestions for a methodical investigation of the nature and chemical composition of the blood. He was also an active participant in the experiments done at Oxford in the 1660s on blood transfusion; several entries in the *Philosophical Transactions of the Royal Society* during the mid-1660s record his thoughts on this subject.

In addition to these works dealing specifically with medical topics, others are crucial to a full understanding of Boyle's medical ideas. One, for example, is *Free Inquiry into the Vulgarly Received Notion of Nature* (1686), in which the concept of the "healing power of nature" is analyzed at length. Boyle's *Disquisition about the Final Causes of Natural Things* (1688) contains his description of the human body as a "hydraulico-pneumatic engine" and is essential to our understanding of the degree to which Boyle perceived the human body as a mechanism. Finally, the second part of *The Christian Virtuoso,* a work that argues why scientific inquiry is a necessary undertaking for the Christian gentleman, clearly delineates the religious motivations at the root of Boyle's scientific perspective.

Clearly, Boyle's medical inquiries were extensive and varied, but behind this variety, I believe, lies a clear vision of medical reform. To begin analyzing Boyle's medical viewpoint and its significance, it is necessary to turn first to an investigation of the initial development of Boyle's medical interest, paying particular attention to the intellectual and religious milieus in which his early work was conducted.

CHAPTER ONE

The Formative Years

To understand the degree of Boyle's interest in medicine and the importance he placed on the pursuit of improvement of human health, it is necessary to know something about the circumstances of Boyle's early life, his personality, his family heritage, his religious beliefs, and his intellectual mentors. All these elements combined to produce in Boyle a strong sense of mission and guidelines for personal conduct that influenced the direction of his thought.

Early Life

Boyle was born at Lismore Castle in southwestern Ireland on 25 January 1626/27, the seventh son and fourteenth of fifteen children of Lady Catherine Fenton and Richard Boyle, the first earl of Cork. His mother died of consumption when Robert Boyle was four, so his recollections of her were few. His father, an ambitious younger son of a family of landed gentry, had achieved success through a combination of talent, good fortune, and considerable guile. He amassed vast wealth, property, and several titles, including that of lord high treasurer of Ireland, while serving in a variety of administrative offices under Elizabeth I, James I, and Charles I. Having elevated his social position, Richard Boyle took great pains to provide for his large family in the manner appropriate to the nobility and to secure (and enhance) his newfound status. He strategically arranged for his daughters to be married off, albeit not many of them happily, to men from other noble families, and for his sons to be provided the broad education then thought proper for English gentlemen. A man of strong religious convictions, including an irenical outlook and an emphatic insistence that Providence had guided (and thus justified) all actions of his life, Richard Boyle actively sought to instill these perspectives in his children as well.[1]

As the youngest son and one whose intellectual gifts were evident from an early age, Robert became (by his own admission) his father's favorite. Introspective in temperament, he was from the outset a serious scholar. He began his formal education at age nine at Eton, where his father's friend Sir Henry Wotton was then provost. He remained there only four years. In October 1639, Robert and his older brother Francis were sent on a grand tour of continental Europe. Noble families of this period typically sent their young sons on extended excursions of this type in order to refine their gentility and to provide a finishing touch to formal education. This cosmopolitan experience was particularly rewarding for Robert, who was inquisitive and creative and hated the rote learning of the schools. This European trip provided him freedom to experience the world and to explore a variety of ideas.

His tutor, mentor, and chaperone for this trip was Isaac Marcombes, of Geneva, who was highly respected by Richard Boyle and who had earlier accompanied Boyle's older brothers Lewis and Roger on their own grand tour. As recent authors have noted, both of the men who had a significant influence on Robert Boyle in his early years, Henry Wotton and Isaac Marcombes, were connected with the irenical Protestant movement, which emphasized the virtues of a unified Protestantism. Boyle's father shared these sentiments.[2] The itinerary followed on Robert Boyle's grand tour, as well as that of the grand tour taken by two of his older brothers, appears to have put the boys in direct contact with other representatives of irenical Protestantism on the Continent.[3] If Richard Boyle's intentions were to inculcate his sons with irenical ideas, then the grand tour served as an excellent vehicle to provide them considerable exposure to those committed to this outlook.

That one important focus of the grand tour was indeed religious instruction is suggested by the tone of the autobiographical fragment the young Robert Boyle wrote not long after returning to England.[4] This autobiographical account describes Boyle's early life at Eton and, more especially, events occurring during the grand tour. It is essentially the story of a religious quest. Boyle portrays himself as particularly preoccupied at that time with theological questions and with his own salvation. To be sure, Boyle wrote this autobiography during the time he was also engaged in writing religious homilies and developing a formal treatise on ethics, and it is possible, therefore, that he may have opted to highlight events of his past that emphasized his religious conversion. Yet the itinerary he followed, which included visits to a great number of religious sites and meetings with individuals holding sophisticated and varied religious outlooks, indicate that the grand tour was designed as much to promote such a religious awakening as to provide an appreciation of continental European culture. In at least Robert's case, the irenical cast of this experience was to have a particularly significant impact, for an irenical perspective was to become an important element both in his science and in his vision of medical reform.

During the grand tour, Boyle developed a very close relationship with Marcombes, whom he describes as sharing with him a commitment to piety and a dislike of pedantry. Even the more unpleasant aspects of Marcombes's personality were appreciated by Boyle, who noted that his tutor's quick temper and his tendency to criticize those whose views he disliked "forc'd him [Boyle] to a very cautious & considerate way of expressing himselfe; which after turn'd to his no small aduantage."[5]

For Robert Boyle and his brother Francis the grand tour was cut short in 1642, when the Great Irish Rebellion caused a dramatic reversal of their father's fortune. Money for their travel expenses now having been cut off, the two young Boyles suddenly found themselves in financial distress. Francis returned to Ireland to fight for the crown, but Robert, who was then only sixteen and in ill health, was invited to return with Marcombes to his home in Geneva. Boyle spent the next two years there, exhausted of his personal funds and subsisting solely upon the generosity of his tutor, and continued his studies.[6]

This unexpected reversal of fortune and the strain of defending his Irish landholdings finally took their toll on Richard Boyle, who died despondent in September 1643. Robert, still devoid of any family financial support and now orphaned as well, was able to return to England only with difficulty. After selling some personal effects, he finally gained passage to England in mid-1644.

Now a young man of eighteen, Boyle found England in the midst of violent civil war, with his own siblings divided in their support of the contending parties. Despite the political and social chaos, Boyle was fortunate in locating in London his older sister Katherine, Lady Ranelagh, whose whereabouts he had not known prior to his arrival from Europe. She was then living at the house of her sister-in-law, Margaret Jones, the wife of Sir John Clotworthy, a leading member of the Presbyterian party in the House of Commons. Lady Ranelagh had gained a considerable reputation as a prominent London hostess by this time and was also well known as a deeply religious Protestant and a strong supporter of the parliamentary cause. She often entertained key members of Parliament at her home. It was fortuitous that Robert went to live with her, for there he became acquainted with men of political influence who secured protection for his estates in England and Ireland and helped him safeguard his inheritance. There also he met men interested in science and in social and religious reform, some of whom were to become close friends and scientific associates.

Sometime during 1645 or 1646, Boyle took up residence at Stalbridge, the country house in Dorsetshire that his father had bequeathed to him. He was to remain there (with frequent trips away, however) until 1655. His introductions to chemistry, atomism, and anatomy all occurred during this period. These were also years of youthful idealism and intense introspection for Boyle. During this time he developed a clear sense of commitment to human improvement and ethical conduct, which both shaped his scientific investigations and served as the foundation of his medical ideas.

The events of Boyle's life at Stalbridge must be viewed against the backdrop of the political, religious, and economic disruption then taking place in England. Having recently suffered through an adolescence punctuated by bouts of religious doubt, personal tragedy, and severe depression, Boyle now had to contend with an unstable political situation in which he saw the fortunes of his family and friends rise and fall. Since they belonged to the newly elevated nobility, the Boyles' status was particularly tenuous, and Robert was forced to travel frequently on missions to safeguard the wealth his father had worked so long to acquire. The political allegiances of his brothers and sisters were split between king and Cromwell, an uncomfortable situation that made Boyle suspect by supporters on each side. Emotional extremism and the divisive rhetoric of religious sectaries were in daily evidence and threatened even further social chaos. Boyle, a quiet, contemplative young man who hated confrontation, clearly found this situation unpleasant.

Boyle coped as best he could during this chaotic period by adopting an overtly unemotional posture. In a letter to Marcombes written in October 1646, he related that he had been arrested briefly and was "forced to observe a very great caution and exact evenness in my carriage . . . it being absolutely necessary for the preservation of a person, whom the unfortunate situation of his fortune made obnoxious to the injuries of both parties, and the protection of neither."[7] Given his dislike of conflict and the real dangers of choosing a losing side in this multidimensional conflict, such a tactic was probably the most wise.

During these years, Boyle developed a strict code of ethics based on personal piety, moderation, and acceptance of Providence.[8] This no doubt provided him a sense of stability lacking in his external environment. Focusing on the providential character of events certainly permitted Boyle to accept the disruptions around him as inevitable, thus freeing him from any obligation of active involvement that the traditional mores of the nobility might have required of him. It is also possible that the sectarian strife then tearing the fabric of his society made Boyle even more receptive to the conciliatory ideas of irenical Protestantism to which he had been exposed during the grand tour.

Despite his attempts to rationalize the circumstances in which he found himself, conditions were stressful, and Boyle, who had never been physically strong, suffered recurrent bouts of illness during these years. His correspondence from the 1640s and early 1650s reveals that he suffered a variety of chills, fevers, and other maladies, which he often undertook to treat on his own. Also at this time, chronic conditions that were to plague him throughout his life, such as kidney stones (of which he first complained as early as 1647) and weakness in his vision, first appeared.

Although Boyle was willing to consult professional physicians for his many and varied ailments, he usually preferred to try to cure himself. He tells us in his autobiographical fragment that this preference for assuming responsibility for his own health care was prompted by a traumatic incident during his Eton days, when he accidentally was given a strong medication meant for someone else and almost lost his life.[9]

Although self-medication and distrust of doctors was hardly unusual in this age,[10] Boyle carried these tendencies to an extreme, becoming a notorious hypochondriac. His family and friends repeatedly complained that he was far too preoccupied with his health. According to the views of the day, they attributed this behavior to his "melancholic temperament." Boyle disputed this, however, maintaining that his melancholy was not the cause but rather the effect of his incessant sickness. In any case, Boyle's reputation for being sickly may have been convenient in distancing him from the political turmoil then sapping the energies of so many of his relatives and compatriots.

Boyle's contemplative nature, the experiences of his grand tour, his revulsion over the social discord in his country, and his preoccupation with his own physical and spiritual health caused him to focus his attention during this period on issues of human morality and ethical conduct. Homiletic writing became his primary activity at Stalbridge. John T. Harwood contends that it was through this authorship that Boyle found a vocation.[11] The significance of this early religious interest to Boyle's mature scientific views and methodology has been recognized by modern scholars.[12] Boyle clearly emphasized that in religion one could find direction and solace from the vicissitudes of everyday life. He held that divine Providence underlay the apparent capriciousness of all temporal events and that a divine order existed beneath the observed variability of natural phenomena. This knowledge allowed the individual to make reasoned, ethical decisions about how to behave in society, even in crisis situations. Boyle's moral stance appears to encompass both an affirmation of social hierarchy and a strong emphasis on piety. While Jacob sees this perspective as related to ideals of social order and an aristocratic ethic, Harwood points out the close similarity between Boyle's views and the values of Christian humanism that developed in the Renaissance.

The first literary project from this period of Boyle's life that receives much mention in his letters to friends and family is his work on ethics, *The Aretology or Ethicall Elements of Robert Boyle.*[13] Boyle's earliest extant letters from Stalbridge include frequent comments about his progress on this treatise. By 1646 he evidently had completed sixteen chapters. Despite its being such a youthful work, it contains the most systematic account of Boyle's ethical position. For our purposes, it is important to recognize that Boyle here expressed views on the ethical basis of the search for knowledge, the centrality of piety and good works, and the rejection of outward display in favor of inner moral constancy that would be incorporated in his mature scientific philosophy.

Boyle's literary output at this time comprised much more than just the work on ethics. In the spring of 1647, Boyle wrote a treatise entitled *Free Discourse against Customary Swearing,* which he dedicated to his sister Joan, countess of Kildare. About this same time he began work on meditative essays that were published much later, in 1665, under the title of *Occasional Reflections.* In 1648 Boyle wrote an essay entitled "On Divinity." His discourse *Some Motives and Incentives to the Love of God* (better known by its running title, *Seraphick Love*) was completed in August 1648. In 1652 he began his "Essay on the Scripture." A list of projected or completed treatises that he compiled in 1649/50 reveals that the majority of his writings were on religion or morals.[14] As a whole, these writings are indicative of a mind coming to grips with what constituted the proper posture for a Christian gentleman in both public and private life.

Boyle's literary efforts repeatedly were hampered by his frequent travel and his chronic ill health. In 1649 he complained to Lady Ranelagh that he had become so weak from a month-long bout of fever that he had been forced to "cast [his] pen into the fire."[15] In November 1651, while attending some festivities near London, he related that he was stricken with "a violent and sudden fitt of Sicknesse, which unfitted me to handle a Pen till God's Blessing vpon a Strange Remedy of a Great Chymist of my Acquaintance restor'd me to Health without the wonted Martyrdome of Physicke."[16]

"Divulging of Useful Truths in Physick"

During this time Boyle developed an avid interest in the preparation of medicinals. This in itself was not unusual, for it was common for learned laymen of the seventeenth century to have some basic knowledge of healing. In rural England especially there existed a tradition of gentry and clergy dispensing remedies in their own communities as an expression of charity. Their service undoubtedly was greatly needed in outlying areas, where medical assistance was less available. Boyle, the country gentleman at Stalbridge, fits into this tradition, but with some important exceptions. His concern for the fragility of his own health and his distrust of physicians tremendously intensified his interest in medical remedies. In addition, Boyle aimed not merely to acquire the usual basic knowledge of herbal cures but to concoct the newer, mineral-based drugs of the iatrochemists in his own laboratory.

Boyle had become fascinated with chemistry quite early, as evidenced by his many frustrated attempts to equip a laboratory at Stalbridge soon after settling there. In a letter to Lady Ranelagh dated 6 March 1646/47, Boyle bemoaned the loss in shipment of "that great earthen furnace, whose conveying hither has taken up so much of my care, and concerning which I made bold very lately to trouble you"; what most exasperated him about this loss was that he had taken such pains "to prevent this furnace the disaster of its predecessors."[17] Boyle would have required such a furnace in order to produce the high heat necessary for operations on metals, and as he notes in this same letter, he had already planned some "fine experiments" that were impeded by the loss of this essential piece of equipment. That he should be willing to try several times to procure this furnace despite the difficulties and expense of transporting it to rural Stalbridge testifies to the seriousness of his desire to pursue chemical activities.

No doubt most of Boyle's initial encouragement in science came from people who frequented Lady Ranelagh's social gatherings. Among these men were two Dutch-born physicians, Arnold and Gerald Boate. In his "Memorials Philosophical for 1649/50" Boyle included some medicinal recipes obtained from these men.[18] The Irish practical chemist Benjamin Worsley, who in 1646 was trying to promote a scheme for the profitable manufacture of saltpeter, was also a member of Lady Ranelagh's social circle. He befriended Boyle quite early and was no doubt the source of much of Boyle's early chemical interest.

From Boyle's early letters and notebooks, it appears that his initial experimental efforts involved the preparation of a wide variety of medicinals. Boyle's interest in developing pharmaceuticals was soon combined with his broader ideas of human improvement and religious reform. By

May 1647, Boyle had completed a treatise that was to be his first published work, outlining the need for free and open communication of medicinal recipes.[19]

The idea that England could take the lead in the reform of Protestantism was prevalent at this time and greatly affected Boyle. Once the ravages of the Thirty Years' War had diminished the probability that continental Europe would retain its leading role in the Protestant Reformation, England was sought out as a more suitable environment for that purpose. Idealistic individuals saw the English civil war as a sign that England would be very responsive to far-reaching social and religious improvements. The future of England was tied to utopian and millenarianist rhetoric hailing the defeat of Antichrist (identified with the Catholic church) and the coming of a new age in which Protestants would unite and share the fruits of their worldly labors for the benefit of all. Many enthusiastically interpreted current events in English politics in providential terms. The promotion of social revolution and educational reform took on the character of a clearly defined religious mission.

A number of recent scholars have attempted to identify specific groups of religious reformers whose programs were particularly influential in stimulating scientific activity; the Puritans have received the most attention.[20] The widespread popularity of ideas such as millenarianism, utilitarianism, and providentialism among all English Protestants, however, makes it difficult to attribute to any single group a key role in promoting science. What *is* important to note is how often social and religious programs encompassed scientific ideas or strategies for technological innovation. Medical reform was also a common theme, especially among those with irenical proclivities who sought new ways to better the human condition.[21]

The Hartlib Circle and the Invisible College

While still at Stalbridge, Boyle became acquainted with the Protestant reformer Samuel Hartlib and forged close ties with many of Hartlib's intellectual associates. The degree to which Hartlib reportedly influenced Boyle's earliest scientific and philosophical perspective has been contested by several modern authors seeking to reevaluate the origins of the Invisible College (which has been identified with the Hartlib circle).

Samuel Hartlib was born in Polish Prussia. His mother was English, and his father had strong English connections. Completing his studies at Cambridge in the mid-1620s, a time when Puritanism was strong there, Hartlib returned to Prussia to find himself in the midst of the turmoil of the Thirty Years' War. Possessed of a powerful and selfless commitment to the idea of a unified Protestantism, Hartlib emigrated to England in 1628, convinced that that nation could become the center of a new united Protestant social order. Because he believed that educational reform was the surest way to achieve social change, he first set up an academy (embodying his own ideas on curricular reform) to teach the sons of noblemen. When this failed, he spent the next thirty years developing and seeking funding (from patrons and the state) for a variety of proposals for the dissemination of knowledge and collective pursuit of science. In his efforts to promote religious and social reform, he drew to his cause not only the divine John Dury but also for a short time the famed educator Jan Amos Comenius, both of whom shared Hartlib's utopian visions.

Hartlib's beliefs for social improvement were couched in terms of the millenarian eschatology so popular in England during this period. Millenarianists held that the Second Coming was near and that the world would soon enter a period in which human welfare would become a predominant theme and all members of society would work together cooperatively for the common good. The knowledge that had been Adam's in the Garden of Eden but had been lost after the Fall would be recovered. Human society would acquire dominion over nature and thereupon use nature's gifts for its own improvement.

To prepare for the coming new age (the year 1666 was widely held to be the date for its inception), Hartlib and his associates urged various programs for centralized collection of information and universal education. Such consolidation of knowledge and training of the knowledge-gatherers would be essential to ensure efficiency in the new world order, when all humankind would work together. An open-minded attitude toward information gathering and information sharing (on an international scale) thus became a salient part of the Hartlib program.

In 1641, believing that the climate in his adopted country was now particularly favorable for implementation of his idealistic programs, Hartlib persuaded the educator and religious reformer Jan Amos Comenius to come to England. He was convinced that those currently in political power would lead the way to the coming enlightenment. Hartlib had already gained the sympathy of several influential members of Parliament for his cause. His main goal at this time was to obtain funding for a collaborative program to disseminate new ideas and encourage the investigation of nature.[22] The outline of this program was articulated in 1641, in the utopian treatise *Macaria,* written by his associate Gabriel Plattes. Plattes hoped by this work to publicize Hartlib's ideas for the benefit of the Long Parliament.[23] *Macaria* combined a utopian message with a set of straightforward proposals for government underwriting of scientific and technological research.

Hartlib was anxious to utilize Comenius's popularity as a religious reformer to gain support for his programs. Comenius espoused a "pansophic" philosophy based on the premise that the fundamental truths underlying all reality could be discovered and exploited for the benefit of all humanity. The reform of language was to be an important part of this effort, since it would make possible universal communication and also provide appropriate terminology for expressing these newly discovered truths.

Hartlib admired not only Comenius's philosophical perspective but the programmatic approach he advocated for attaining the goals of universal peace and prosperity. Comenius emphasized that true piety is best expressed through information sharing and the dedication of one's public life to the enhancement of human welfare. This is basically a Calvinistic perspective, but with a decidedly Baconian emphasis, since Comenius focused on science and education as the rallying points around which to base these communal efforts.[24]

Although Hartlib optimistically expected that his reform proposals would finally be implemented in 1641, his hopes dimmed when England succumbed to civil war the next year and Hartlib's former supporters in the government turned their attention to more immediate political needs. Given this change in the intellectual climate, Comenius soon abandoned England for Europe. His pansophic perspective, however, remained an integral part of the Hartlib program.

Even before civil war broke out, Hartlib had begun to draw to him a wide variety of individuals who he felt could further his reform goals. In response to the altered political and social situation, Hartlib now promoted himself and his "circle" of associates not only as leaders of spiritual and educational reform but as advocates for practical scientific researches that could have immediate benefit. This change represents more a pragmatic strategy to retain political patronage than any conceptual shift, since Hartlib's ultimate goals of broad social and religious reform remained intact.

Hartlib gradually became a mentor to a large group of inventors, chemists, and "agriculturalists," most of them strongly committed to the Baconian experimental agenda. Some shared his larger vision of disseminating scientific ideas for the greater benefit of society. Others were more interested in exploiting new scientific and technological innovations for personal profit. Hartlib, with his eclectic perspective and commitment to a unified society, was willing to patronize anyone who could further his schemes of amassing and disseminating useful knowledge, whatever their ultimate motives might be. He sought financial support from prominent members of Parliament with widely differing political outlooks. True to his utopian ideal of an improved social order, Hartlib was willing to show by personal example that a variety of philosophical, political, and even educational outlooks could be subsumed within his broad program of cooperative enterprise.

At this time, Hartlib cultivated an extensive correspondence with intellectuals on the Continent, becoming eventually a one-man clearinghouse for the international dissemination of scientific information. His ability to act as a facilitator of communication between men of widely different interests and perspectives and his optimistic belief in human progress were to prove extremely attractive to idealistic young men such as Robert Boyle.

The first extant letter from Boyle to Hartlib is dated April 1646/47, several years after Boyle returned to England from his grand tour. The relatively late date of this letter has been used as evidence that Hartlib could not have been influential in the initial development of Boyle's scientific and social outlook;[25] however, this does not necessarily suggest that they did not know of each other before then. It is clear that Lady Ranelagh was acquainted with Hartlib earlier than this, for her relative Dorothy Moore (who had married Hartlib's close colleague John Dury in 1645) wrote to her in February 1645 asking her to influence her important friends in Parliament to provide Hartlib with financial support.[26] Writing of Boyle's acquaintances after his return to London from the grand tour, his modern biographer, R. E. W. Maddison, suggests that Hartlib had by this time been known to Lady Ranelagh, Dorothy Moore Dury, and Sir John Clotworthy and his wife Margaret "for some years" and thus probably was known to Robert Boyle at quite an early date. John Harwood, in his recent investigation of Boyle's ethical writings, notes that while Boyle was still in Geneva with Marcombes, Lady Ranelagh was "actively supporting Dury and Hartlib, so much so that it was common for Hartlib's mail to be delivered to her home or to Sir John Clotworthy's."[27] Since Lady Ranelagh was instrumental in introducing Boyle to so many of her intellectual associates at this time, it seems plausible that Hartlib would have been among them, especially since she was familiar with and supportive of his reform program. At the very least, Lady Ranelagh, possessed of the same irenical perspective as her young brother, would have informed Boyle of Hartlib's spiritual reform agenda.[28]

Once the two men became acquainted, Hartlib played a significant role in encouraging Boyle's efforts and brought him into his own circle of associates. Most of Boyle's closest colleagues during the time prior to his move to Oxford in 1655—Worsley, the Boate brothers, the chemists George Starkey and Frederick Clodius (Hartlib's son-in-law), the inventor-physician William Petty, and the alchemist and mechanical philosopher Kenelm Digby—were all members of the Hartlib circle, and some of them were first introduced to Boyle by Hartlib. Through his fairly regular correspondence with Boyle during the years Boyle lived at Stalbridge, Hartlib also provided information about the activities of scientific groups on the Continent, keeping Boyle abreast of the newest ideas, projects, and publications and suggesting people for Boyle to contact in his travels. Hartlib's willingness to serve as a conduit of scientific information permitted Boyle, despite the disruptions so prevalent during these years, to keep well informed about new inventions and experiments and to become acquainted with men engaged in a variety of scientific investigations. This resulted in further broadening Boyle's own scientific interests. In return for his attentiveness to Boyle's scientific education, Hartlib gained in Boyle a young, enthusiastic, wealthy, and influential sympathizer whose family's contacts with influential members of Parliament held the promise of aid to Hartlib's utopian cause.

Improvement of human health was a specific focus of Hartlib's overall effort. The outline of such a program was articulated in *Macaria,* where the need for the government to concern itself with public health was advocated specifically. The treatise describes a utopian world in which a government-sponsored scientific "college" engaged in medical investigation as one of its primary goals: "They have an house, or Colledge of experience, where they deliver out yeerly such medicines as they find out by experience; and all such as shall be able to demonstrate any experiment for the health or wealth of men, are honourably rewarded at the publicke charge, by which their skill in Husbandry, Physick, and Surgerie, is most excellent."[29]

Programs such as Hartlib's, which related scientific activity specifically to good works, must have been very appealing to Boyle. Given Boyle's concern with moral rectitude and godliness, a religious justification particularly for engaging in chemical activity would have been significant in mollifying any moral qualms Boyle may have had about involving himself in work that was commonly associated with esoteric magic and the greed of the alchemist.[30] His concern for the improvement of medicine, based on his own distrust of physicians and his interest in developing his own drugs, would also have led him to an appreciation of Hartlib's vision of collaborative pharmaceutical research and free sharing of medicinal recipes.

"Divulging of Useful Truths in Physick"

Although the utopian vision of a state-funded "college" engaged in scientific research did not come to fruition, in 1646 Hartlib attempted to interest Parliament in funding a more modest Office of Address, an agency with two departments: the Office of Address for Communications would accumulate information on new inventions and new ideas on an international scale; the Office of Address for Accommodations would serve as a labor exchange. The goals of the Office of Address were at least as lofty as those of the "college of experience" in *Macaria.* In both the notion of bringing people together to share and assess information is paramount. As Webster points out, the design of the Office of Address, like that of the "college" in *Macaria,* had utopian overtones.[31]

It was during these years when Hartlib and others were actively promoting the Office of Address that Boyle wrote a letter to his old tutor Marcombes relating that in addition to his treatise on ethics, "the other humane studies I apply myself to, are natural philosophy, the mechanics, and husbandry, according to the principles of our new philosophical college, that values no knowledge but as it hath a tendency to use."[32] He then goes on to ask Marcombes for information regarding husbandry practices in his locale. This letter is dated 22 October 1646.

A letter to Francis Tallents written slightly later, in February 1647, describes the character of the scientific investigators of this college in especially laudatory terms:

> The corner-stones of the invisible, or (as they term themselves) the philosophical college, do now and then honour me with their company. . . . men of so capacious and searching spirits, that school-philosophy is but the lowest region of their knowledge; and yet, though ambitious to lead the way to any generous design, of so humble and teachable a genius, as they disdain not to be directed to the meanest, so he can but plead reason for his opinion; persons that endeavour to put narrow-mindedness out of countenance, by the practice of so extensive a charity, that it reaches unto everything called man.[33]

The composition of the Invisible College has long been a topic of speculation. A major problem is the lack of specific evidence concerning its membership or of the degree of Boyle's direct participation in it.[34] Although Thomas Birch associated the Invisible College with those virtuosi meeting to discuss new scientific ideas at Gresham College in London and Oxford in the mid-1640s, arguments have been posed against this thesis.[35] An alternate view associates the Invisible College with members of the Hartlib circle, either exclusively or in conjunction with the Gresham Group. This idea has been challenged as well.[36] A recent reinterpretation has been forwarded by Charles Webster and Nicholas Canny, who identify the inspiration for the Invisible College with that group of Anglo-Irish émigrés who were part of Lady Ranelagh's circle in London at the time Boyle returned from his grand tour.

Webster asserts that Hartlib himself was not a founding member of the Invisible College, since it was in existence before Boyle met Hartlib. His argument is based on the late date of the first extant letter from Boyle to Hartlib and a highly idiosyncratic interpretation of other (dated and undated) extant letters, from which he concludes that the Invisible College refers to an association of Anglo-Irish émigrés, led by Boyle and Benjamin Worsley, formed for the specific purpose of devising scientific schemes for the profitable exploitation of resources in Ireland. Webster suggests that many of the projects Boyle's associates (including Worsley and the Boate brothers) were engaged in at this time had a clearly Irish focus. However, he concludes that once Hartlib was informed of the Invisible College by Boyle, the activities of that college were absorbed under the broader umbrella of Hartlib's Office of Address.

Canny also argues that the Anglo-Irish refugees in London had a long-standing, active agenda aimed at reforming (Anglicizing) Irish society via economic and technological improvements and that although Hartlib's rhetoric "sharpened" their perceptions, he was not the initial inspiration for them. Canny sees in Richard Boyle an exemplar of one who encouraged profitable initiatives to exploit Ireland's natural resources and notes that Robert Boyle's views on the practical benefits of science stem from this source.

Although the views of Webster and Canny serve as a useful corrective to monocausal theories of the rise of utilitarian science and shed light on the aims of the Anglo-Irish, arguments identifying the circle of Anglo-Irish planters as originators of the Invisible College and especially the suggestion that Boyle led this group are not wholly convincing. Webster's thesis can only be tenable if one accepts his chronology, but this is based on a highly speculative interpretation of references, authorship, and (where dates are not known) dating of extant letters between Boyle and Worsley and Boyle and Hartlib and on the assumption that Boyle was unacquainted with Hartlib before 1645. It is also puzzling why the still quite young, idealistic Boyle (who sought to distance himself from the political scene and whose long absence from both England and Ireland could hardly have made him much aware of the economic potentials of cultivating natural resources of either country) would be willing or capable of leadership (or even accepted as a leader) in an enterprise that might be best described as venture capitalism. In the 1647 letter to Francis Tallents,

Boyle refers to the "corner-stones" of the Invisible College "now and then honour[ing] me with their company." This hardly suggests that Boyle was a leader of this group. Further, would Boyle have written so glowingly of the Invisible College if it had a primarily profit-making focus, even if it was couched in the rhetoric of "improving" Ireland?

Given what we know of Boyle's strict, almost ascetic sense of proper Christian behavior, his desire to keep a low profile in this politically difficult period, and his altruism, it does not seem plausible that Boyle would be very interested in leading a group with such provincial and materialist aims, much less expounding its virtues to Marcombes, the mentor and confidant he so respected. Canny argues that the main goal of the Hartlib program was control of nature and technological progress and that since this was equally characteristic of the Anglo-Irish group, that latter circle was at least as influential as Hartlib in shaping Boyle's scientific outlook. However, control over nature was a common rallying point for empirical science in that age—stemming ultimately from the Hermetic tradition and Renaissance natural magic. In fact, Carolyn Merchant has highlighted this theme as central to the period and has indicated how it affected broader social perceptions, such as gender.[37] This cannot be called the defining characteristic of Hartlib's group; it is far more accurate to point to the broad-minded, altruistic aspects of Hartlib's program. Boyle would have found such an idealistic focus, emphasizing cooperation, social and religious harmony, and human improvement, including improvements in health, much more compelling than successful technological "control" over natural resources.

Unless additional hard evidence turns up, it will never be possible to ascertain the composition of the Invisible College definitively. The problem is compounded by the fact that a number of proposals for collaborative research—some with a purely practical profit-seeking goals, others with mystical or occult overtones—were forwarded during this period. The Invisible College could probably be identified with a fair number of these. All that is certain is that Boyle particularly admired the Invisible College for the intellectual integrity and altruism of its participants and for its potential for creating a better society. This seems clear in the comments Boyle provides in the few extant letters that specifically refer to the Invisible College. In the letters to Marcombes and Tallents, it is the potential for amassing practical knowledge and the open-minded and multifaceted approach to the investigation of nature exhibited by members of the Invisible College that he praises most.

The advent of the Office of Address so close to the time Boyle writes about the Invisible College, the similarities between Boyle's irenical views and those of Hartlib, and the eclecticism and desire to rise above special interests shared by both men make a connection between the Invisible College and the activities of the Hartlib circle very plausible. Webster, of course, argues an eventual connection between the Invisible College and the Office of Address but sees it only as a second stage in the evolution of the profit-oriented Irish group founded earlier by Boyle and Worsley.

If one accepts the idea that Hartlib's proposal for the Office of Address still retained much of his earlier utopian vision, something Webster himself admits, then it can be argued that Hartlib was very consistent in his purpose during the years he promoted his ideas, scaling down his proposals in response to his realistic assessments of the availability of funding but never losing sight of what he wished ultimately to achieve. Despite the diversity of those in his circle, the Hartlib group as a whole conveyed views that were distinctive and recognizable to outsiders. They were perceived as social reformers aiming to disseminate knowledge and improve human welfare. Boyle would doubtless have known this, even before any formal funding for the Office of Address was obtained. For his part, Hartlib, or indeed any of his followers, would have been more than happy to encourage Boyle's participation. Despite the lack of concrete evidence, it is not implausible to suggest that Boyle's references to the Invisible College most likely fit the description of the activities (formalized and funded or not) of members of the Hartlib group.

Early Iatrochemical Interests

Boyle's own scientific work at this time, as I have noted, was focused largely on the chemical preparation of medicinals. Letters written in this period frequently mention his attempts to acquire recipes from others, despite a reluctance on the part of many to divulge recipes they wished to keep secret. The desire for secrecy was common among chemists not only because of the traditional esotericism of alchemy but for practical reasons, since a person could gain considerable reputation and wealth from maintaining exclusive control over the production and dispensing of a secret recipe.

In 1647, about the time he was praising the activities of the Invisible College to Tallents, Boyle wrote a treatise on the free communication of medicinal recipes. This treatise, "An Epistolical Discourse of Philaretus to Empericus, inviting all true lovers of Vertue and Mankind, to a free and generous Communication of their Secrets and Receipts in Physick," was published anonymously in 1655 in a compendium of works by several authors entitled *Chymical, Medicinal, and Chyrurgical Addresses made to*

S. Hartlib.[38] It was Boyle's first publication. The tone of this discourse is clearly in keeping both with Boyle's own moral convictions and with the aims of the Hartlib circle and, ultimately, with the utopian message of *Macaria:* that free communication of drug discoveries should be encouraged as an act of Christian charity. Boyle argued that these discoveries for the improvement of human health are ultimately a revelation of God. The developers of such recipes are thereby "stewards of God's grace" and thus have a religious duty to communicate this revealed knowledge to their fellows for the good of all humanity. To withhold such information for personal profit is unethical.

This small treatise is also revealing of Boyle's general attitudes toward medicine as a developing body of knowledge and toward proper scientific method, which he was to articulate more clearly during the course of his life. The cooperative nature of scientific activity, the need for verification of reported results, the benefits to humankind of properly conducted science, and the idea that the scientist in seeking to procure and communicate knowledge of nature is engaging in a religious quest are all evident themes in this short work.

Boyle's personal skill in chemistry grew rapidly at this time. As I have noted, his first chemical investigations were conducted during times when he was too ill or too distracted to write, but chemical experimentation soon became a consuming fascination. By 1649 Boyle wrote his sister: "Vulcan has so transported and bewitched me, that as the delights I taste in it make me fancy my laboratory a kind of Elysium, so as if the threshold of it possessed the quality the poets ascribed to that Lethe, their fictions made men taste of before their entrance into those seats of bliss, I there forget my standish and my books, and almost all things."[39]

At this same time, the Hartlib group was becoming more and more infused with individuals interested in iatrochemistry. The first English translation of the works of Van Helmont in 1648 had revived interest in the chemical philosophy, and this led to new works by iatrochemists and new translations of Paracelsus. The earlier practice among the English of integrating iatrochemical remedies into the pharmacopoeia without changing the essentials of the prevailing Galenic theory was seen as no longer tenable; a better understanding of the Paracelsian and Helmontian ideas on nature made proponents of these views call for nothing less than a new medical philosophy based on chemistry.[40] Like Paracelsus, many English and continental iatrochemists believed that nature's most basic secrets would be revealed ultimately through an understanding of chemical composition. To this end they urged the establishment of chemical laboratories both to extend knowledge and to discover new and profitable medicinal remedies. These individuals found Hartlib's schemes for educational reform and his support of innovative scientific activity especially appealing.

After 1648 a number of iatrochemists joined the Hartlib circle. Many of these men were German Protestants who had seen religious reform efforts in their own country thwarted by the outcome of the Thirty Years' War and who hoped that with the establishment of the English Commonwealth Hartlib's utopian schemes, which gave legitimacy to their endeavors, would have a greater chance for success.[41] The entry of skilled iatrochemists into the Hartlib circle was significant, for these men provided opportunities for experimental collaboration and turned Hartlib's attention more and more toward projects for private or public funding of chemical pursuits.

By the early 1650s, Boyle's extant lists, such as the "Memorialls Philosophicall of 1651/52" and the "Philosophical Diary of January 1654/55," reveal a broad acquaintance with remedies in vogue among the iatrochemists.[42] One of Boyle's favorite recipes was the *ens veneris,* prepared from calcined vitriol and used for a variety of ailments, which he had perfected with the collaboration of the Helmontian iatrochemist and Hartlib associate George Starkey.[43]

Hartlib's iatrochemist colleagues set up a number of private laboratories in and around London in the early 1650s. In 1654 Hartlib wrote Boyle that a Chemical Council had been established near his home at Charing Cross. This was possibly a clearinghouse for iatrochemical discoveries and information coming from these many separate laboratories. Peter Elmer has pointed out that support for this Chemical Council came from those imbued with irenical ideas.[44] Significantly, it was at the height of activity of this Chemical Council, in 1655, that Hartlib's *Chymical, Medicinal, and Chyrurgical Addresses* first appeared.

Many then thought that the best way to coordinate the activities of the iatrochemists would be to establish a nationally sponsored "universal laboratory." Just such a laboratory had been envisioned in *Macaria.* Financing for such a national effort, however, was not forthcoming. Therefore, in 1654 Sir Kenelm Digby initiated a plan to establish a "universal laboratory" as a private endowment.

Digby, a Royalist and rehabilitated Catholic who also had a family connection to Boyle, operated on the fringes of the Hartlib group. He had spent his time during the years of English civil war in exile in France, but he returned to England in 1654 in an attempt to retrieve his landholdings, which had been sequestered by Cromwell. While in England, he became very impressed with the chemical work being done by Hartlib's son-in-law, Frederick Clodius, whose lab was then in Hartlib's kitchen. Digby proposed that Clodius become his partner in establishing a "universal laboratory," a venture toward which Digby was willing to contribute the sum of six hundred to seven hundred pounds once he had successfully recovered his lost property. The proposition was appealing, but Clodius and Hartlib viewed Digby's motives as somewhat suspect. After all, his Catholic sympathies made Digby an unusual ally in the quest for Protestant unity. Clodius, like Hartlib, was well acquainted with Boyle at this time, and since Boyle knew of Digby's work, Clodius solicited Boyle's advice on whether to proceed with this project.

Boyle's answer is not known, but he was soon to return to England from an extended trip to Ireland and may well have decided to lend his support to this project in some way, for there is evidence of substantial contact between Boyle, Digby, and Clodius after Boyle's return to England. Boyle had been aware of Digby's serious interests in science before this time and had acquired a familiarity with Digby's atomistic views, which he cited in the draft of an early unpublished treatise, "Of ye Atomicall Philosophy," written about 1650. There he, like Digby, equates atoms with minima, which had chemical properties and maintained their unique qualities in chemical reactions. He may also have been acquainted with Digby's alchemical interests and with his mechanistic interpretation of the "powder of sympathy," a variant of the "weapon salve" devised by Paracelsus, which involved the cure of wounds at a distance. References to Digby in Boyle's writings became much more frequent after 1654. Boyle's "Philosophical Diary" for January–February 1655 lists chemical information and recipes received from Digby, Clodius, and others, and his "Promiscuous Observations" for 24 September 1655 cites Digby even more often.[45] Boyle's unpublished work entitled "Reflexions on the Experiments vulgarly alledged to evince the 4 Peripatetique Elements, or ye 3 Chymicall Principles of Mixt Bodies," which Marie Boas Hall sees as an early version of *The Sceptical Chymist* and dates as 1654/55, cites Digby almost exclusively.[46] It thus appears that Digby, Boyle, and Clodius were all in close communication during the time plans were forwarded to establish the privately funded "universal laboratory."

Whether this laboratory ever became a physical reality as it was originally planned is questionable, for Digby, Boyle, and Clodius soon went separate ways. Boyle relocated to Oxford at the end of 1655 or early 1656. Digby returned to France in 1656 and became involved in scientific activity there. He maintained correspondence, nonetheless, with both Boyle and Clodius.[47] Clodius may have continued to develop plans for the laboratory on his own, but his financial situation was poor, and he could not have launched such a project without significant monetary backing. In a letter to Boyle dated 14 September 1658, Hartlib commented:

> [Clodius] wrote to you last Saturday. His chemical college or laboratory will not be so much prostituted as you fear; but there was an absolute necessity to resolve upon such a course amongst a few confiding friends. There are near three furnaces finished, but five more must be added unto them; and having these, they shall be able to command any kind of operation whatsoever.[48]

This would indicate that Clodius was involved with the establishment of a laboratory several years after his initial contact with Digby. A clue to the purpose of this laboratory is provided in this same letter, when Hartlib informs Boyle that a "like charitable design . . . a charitable . . . laboratory for the poor" is to be founded at Durham.[49] Such aims would be in keeping with the interest of Protestant reformers in general and Hartlib in particular in tying research programs to social welfare.[50] Boyle's concern for the success of this venture is evident in his letter of September 14. Further evidence that Boyle may have taken a personal interest in Clodius's laboratory is provided by a letter to Boyle from Johann Christian Agricola, written in April 1668, which refers to Agricola's having waited upon Boyle in Clodius's laboratory "almost ten years ago," that is, in 1658.[51] And in a letter of 1663, Clodius requests additional financial assistance from Boyle.[52] The purpose of this assistance is unclear, but the letter certainly indicates that Boyle had continued to support Clodius's work. If Clodius's effort was indeed aimed at setting up a laboratory for the benefit of the poor, it would be logical for Boyle to be interested in it, since such an endeavor would have been consistent with his general interest in promoting scientific projects that would benefit society.

Boyle's keen interest in the chemical preparation of medicinals and his friendship with many iatrochemists in this period bears closer examination. To what extent did Boyle incorporate the philosophical ideas underlying iatrochemistry, based on the metaphor of the world as a giant chemical retort, on the existing occult correspondences between natural objects, and on the categorization of matter in terms of a few dynamic principles rather than the traditional four elements?[53] The link between iatrochemistry and irenical Protestantism noted by Elmer indicates that Boyle would be receptive, at least initially, to viewing nature in chemical terms.[54] Certainly Boyle, like many others at this time, had become quite knowledgeable about the theories of Paracelsus and Van Helmont.[55] We know that Boyle collaborated very closely with several iatrochemists of the Hartlib circle and that he very probably gave at least one of them, Clodius, financial backing. The Helmontian chemist George Starkey, another member of the Hartlib circle and the person who worked with Boyle to develop the *ens veneris,* not only dedicated a major work to Boyle but referred to him as an avid Helmontian.[56]

Allen Debus has suggested that Boyle had accepted some aspects of Van Helmont's ideas at this time but that he then abandoned this focus once he took up residence at Oxford in 1655 and began to develop his corpuscular philosophy.[57] From comments made in Boyle's published writings, however, it appears that he was always extremely cautious about what to accept from both Paracelsus and Van Helmont. For example, he never agreed with the more mystical and occult interpretations of chemical action espoused in the Paracelsian and Helmontian philosophy, preferring always a material view. In fact, the removal of occult explanations from science was to become one of Boyle's major goals. Many iatrochemists did not share this view, however. If anything, buoyed by the new availability of Helmontian writings, English iatrochemists became even more enamored of theories based on occult correspondences and the existence of spiritual forces in nature. Those who forwarded such theories found themselves supported by the more radical Protestant sects, whose notions of religious enthusiasm fit well with the iatrochemists' own emphasis on divine inspiration as the source of all knowledge. Boyle, whose moderate views were opposed to the radical sectaries (and who especially feared the unbridled excesses of religious enthusiasm), may well have wished to distance himself from this particular aspect of iatrochemical thought.[58]

This does not mean, however, that he abandoned all concepts he acquired from the study of the chemical philosophers. We should not assume that Boyle considered the work of Paracelsians and Helmontians in its totality and then rejected it; it may be more accurate to suggest that Boyle considered Paracelsian and Helmontian thought as a body of knowledge containing both practical and philosophical aspects that he absorbed in his youth, selected from and modified throughout his life, and integrated where appropriate into his mature philosophy. Nor is it necessary to assume that Boyle's atomist leanings would preclude his admitting Paracelsian or Helmontian conceptualizations of nature. As John Henry points out, "It was perfectly possible to amalgamate atomist heuristic with . . . Paracelsian/Helmontian world views."[59]

Although Boyle accepted the Paracelsian notion that reading the Book of Nature was a means of venerating God and that God would reward investigators by permitting them to discover useful remedies in nature, he denied that God would bestow this knowledge by divine illumination. In Boyle's interpretation, God did not target certain "adepts" and then reveal to them, and them alone, divine Truths; rather, he assisted and encouraged the labors of all pious researchers by rewarding their collaborative labor with gradual insights into the workings of nature. The study of nature, then, for Boyle involved a specific procedural strategy, which, as Jacob notes, was associated with that "reason and industry" necessary to "make and keep men virtuous."[60] To implement such a strategy, long-term collaboration was imperative. Directing one's labors toward reading the Book of Nature was a means of avoiding idleness, which could lead to sin. The rationale for engaging in such labor was that important knowledge would be gained by these efforts. God would bless the quest, but he would not permit shortcuts to truth.

Boyle emphasized that such knowledge, once obtained, should not be kept secret. Once revealed publicly, any new useful information could immediately be widely disseminated, and this would best benefit society as a whole. Perhaps Boyle was moved to take a strong stand against esoteric knowledge because chemical work especially had traditionally been associated with secret information and dabbling in the forbidden. Boyle was especially aware of this, and as Hunter points out, it troubled him.[61] By making open sharing of iatrochemical findings a part of his social agenda, Boyle avoided any impression that what he was doing was in any way questionable. On the contrary, he showed that there was a place for legitimate chemical activity openly conducted, which would not threaten the social system, as esoteric alchemy was suspected of doing. Such activity, in fact, would be a moral act in that society would benefit. He thus fully separates iatrochemical pursuits from the traditional mystique of alchemy (and its later association with religious enthusiasm) and makes iatrochemistry a part of public science in the Baconian tradition.

Boyle also agreed with the idea common among iatrochemists that by investigating nature one could see clearly the truth of a preordained world order in which all things were interrelated. Usually articulated in terms of macrocosm-microcosm correspondences, this view of the interrelatedness of all substances in nature underlay much iatrochemical interpretation and was seen as consistent with theological notions of Divine Design.

From a purely medical perspective it is also significant that Boyle's position differed from that of those Helmontians who held that no accommodation between Helmontian and older Galenic ideas was possible and who essentially urged a revolution in medical thought in which Galenism would be discarded in favor of iatrochemical theories and methods. As we shall see, Boyle wanted any Galenic ideas still valid to be accepted along with the newer iatrochemical ones. He made it quite clear, in fact, that advancement in medicine was possible only through the unification of existing concepts and practical discoveries and that this goal was not well served by the current fragmentation of medicine into special interest groups espousing competing theories.

The Crisis in English Medicine in Boyle's Day

The fragmentation of medical practice in mid-seventeenth-century England was extensive. The growing demand for health care during the early part of the century had led to a proliferation of a great variety of practitioners who lacked formal university training. This produced a crisis within the medical profession that became prominent at precisely the time when Boyle was beginning to develop his scientific thought.

Medicine had become professionalized by the end of the medieval period, with university training becoming the distinguishing mark of the medical professional.[62] Learned medicine thereafter set the standards for medical practice. Once in control of its educational base, university-trained physicians were able to extend their control to the regulation of medical practice in the community.

Traditionally, the universities had emphasized speculative studies, with just enough vocational emphasis to "fit the student for the task he was to perform." This was as true for the curriculum in theology or law as in for that in medicine. However, as Vern Bullough suggests, because medicine lacked the "intellectual prestige of theology or the opportunities for advancement found in law," in order to maintain its professional image, "the physicians had to sacrifice some of their less intellectual aspects, particularly manipulative techniques."[63] This created a gulf between physicians and surgeons, with surgeons being assigned a lower place in the medical hierarchy. Still lower were barbers (who gradually encroached upon the surgeon's domain) and a wide range of empirics (many of whom specialized in one type of medical treatment) and outright quacks.

This separation between the various groups of medical practitioners continued into the seventeenth century. In England, where the university medical faculties were not as powerful as elsewhere, the Royal College of Physicians was established in 1518 to serve as an agency for regulating the profession. Harold Cook notes that it also served to "encourage medical learning, to tap the advice of learned men, and probably, to create a network of patronage for physicians close to the [royal] court." Comprising university-educated physicians and sponsored by the crown, the college set standards for the medical profession in England. As Cook points out, the maintenance of the "dignity and supremacy" of university-based learning became a primary goal of the college, even more so in the face of increasing economic and social insecurities caused by proliferating numbers of competitors in the medical marketplace.[64]

The college both encouraged medical learning "by emulation" and attempted (with varying success) to regulate the licensing of practitioners in London.[65] In 1523 a parliamentary act extended this licensing power to all of England, which heightened the stature of the college but was for practical purposes unenforceable (and thus ignored).[66]

The Royal College retained its public image as a learned society into the seventeenth century, but as Cook notes, it became subject to all the "political and social vicissitudes" of that century. The increase in the population of London rendered greater opportunities for medical practice and profit, challenging the college's regulatory capabilities. New "intellectual innovations" competed with old traditions, and as a learned society the college was expected to pass judgment on these.

It was difficult for the college to respond to these challenges, especially when political changes in the mid-seventeenth century threatened their support base.[67] By mid-century, prosecution of unlicensed practitioners had become uneven at best, partly because the college, desperate to maintain its corporate power in the face of the political turmoil of the 1640s and 1650s, had assumed a strategy of accommodation to whatever political forces currently held power. Even when the college had the energy to exercise control over unlicensed practitioners, it was sometimes politically inexpedient to do so. In the years just prior to and during the English civil war, the Royal College of Physicians faced open attack by both disenfranchised practitioners and its current political enemies for its monopolistic practices and philosophical conservatism.

The activities of the Royal College were by no means as reactionary as some critics maintained. As the college lost the ability to regulate medical practice—its primary purpose—it turned more and more to justifying itself as a formal learned society.[68] Thus during the interregnum and early Restoration the college encouraged researches that would incorporate new ideas into the traditional academic framework of Galenism. The establishment of a museum and library at the college, funded by William Harvey, enabled the members to collaborate on anatomical work. Chemical remedies, which had been gradually incorporated into the national pharmacopoeia since the early seventeenth century, were being formally evaluated and discussed by the college membership.[69]

"Divulging of Useful Truths in Physick"

In 1651, however, the chemical reformer Noah Biggs published a particularly vituperative attack on the college under the title *The Vanity of the Craft of Physick*.[70] Biggs called for the rejection of the traditional academic foundation of medicine and its replacement with one based on Helmontian principles. Biggs's position was shared by a growing number of other iatrochemists in this period. This extremism was seen as particularly threatening by the college, which had been willing to incorporate new ideas but was wholly opposed to abandoning the (Galenic) academic base on which its legitimacy so obviously rested. Of most concern was the threat of medical reform enthusiasts to the conventional hierarchical structure of the profession.

It was at about this time (1647–49) that Boyle began to draft a work that would be published in 1663 as *Considerations Touching the Usefulness of Experimental Natural Philosophy, Part I.* This work sets forth Boyle's most specific suggestions concerning how a broad experimental program could improve medicine. Members of the Royal College of Physicians were among those Boyle most hoped to persuade with his arguments on how his experimental methodology and theoretical outlook could promote medical reform. Boyle maintained that learned physicians need not wholly abandon their traditional ideas (most of which were based on Galen), because of the continued value of some of these time-honored notions and also, most likely, because he too saw a threat to the social order if medicine as a discipline were to become deregulated. His goal was to strengthen medicine as a profession, not to destroy the foundations on which it rested.

Boyle's commitment to compromise and tolerance in all levels of human activity and his aversion to sectarianism, particularly in its radical forms, also influenced his views on how medical reform could be accomplished peacefully. Just as his agenda for religious reform focused on Protestant unity, so his medical agenda came to be based on the idea that a synthesis of medical thought held the best hope for true advancement in human health. Insofar as the iatrochemists could add their insights into the cause and cure of disease, Boyle was in favor of them; he would not, however, support any efforts by the more radical iatrochemists or other critics of the status quo to overthrow the existing medical framework and polarize the medical community.

Boyle shared with the English physician Thomas Sydenham a vision of the physician's moral duty to improve medicine. Andrew Cunningham notes that for Sydenham this notion had political overtones, stemming from a Hartlib agenda that placed the hopes of millenarian Protestants on the "Commonwealth men" in power in the 1650s and assumed that the leaders in the coming new order would be members of the educated gentry.[71] It was clearly the professional physician that Sydenham urged to set the moral example, not unlicensed empirics. Given what we know of Boyle's emphasis on proper moral conduct for the Christian gentleman, a topic thoroughly addressed by Jacob,[72] and Boyle's respect for the traditional social order, it is apparent that his attitude was similar. Furthermore, it probably stemmed from the same Hartlibian influence.

Anatomy, Physiology, and Mechanism

Boyle's specific researches in medicine in this Stalbridge period extended beyond his work in chemistry and his consideration of iatrochemical views of physiological processes. Other medical men introduced him to additional areas of medical investigation and influenced the direction of his medical thought. Two such individuals were Nathaniel Highmore and William Petty.

From Nathaniel Highmore, a physician who practiced at Sherborne, near Stalbridge, Boyle gained a knowledge of anatomy and physiology,[73] an appreciation of the usefulness of the microscope as a tool for observing organic structure, and an idea of how biological operations could be described in mechanistic terms.

Highmore had received his medical degree at Oxford in 1642. While there, he had become one of a small group of scientists collaborating with William Harvey.[74] Highmore and Harvey at that time conducted joint experiments in embryology. In 1651 Highmore published two major works. The first, *Corporis humani disquisitio anatomica in qua sanguinis circulationem prosecutus est,* was dedicated to Harvey. It was the first systematic anatomical textbook to recognize the circulation of the blood and was long considered a standard textbook.[75] Robert Frank has pointed out that Highmore's interpretations are far more mechanistic than those of Harvey.[76] Highmore's views on the particulate nature of the blood were extremely similar to those Boyle posited in his own later medical writing.

Highmore's second 1651 publication, *The History of Generation,* was apparently the result of his earlier joint embryological work with Harvey.[77] Highmore here gave an atomistic explanation of embryological development. To this work was appended "Discourse of the Cure of Wounds by Sympathy," which described in atomistic terms the efficacy of healing agents that worked at a distance, such as the "powder of sympathy" and "weapon salve."[78] This work was dedicated to Boyle; in fact, it was the first work ever dedicated to him.

"Divulging of Useful Truths in Physick"

The association of Boyle's name with this work is significant for two reasons. It not only indicates a close association between Boyle and Highmore and suggests that Highmore may have played a role in Boyle's initial experimentation in anatomy and physiology but also links Boyle to those seeking mechanistic interpretations of nature.

We know that Boyle was interested in atomistic ideas as well as chemical ones by this time. References to Pierre Gassendi in Boyle's writings make it clear that he was particularly well acquainted with Gassendi's work, which focused largely on articulating atomistic ideas in a form palatable to Christian theology. Gassendi's ability to make atomism an acceptable subject of study for Christians would have given Boyle the security that he could investigate such ideas for himself in good conscience, a matter of no small concern to him.[79]

In an early work, "Of ye Atomicall Philosophy," which is probably the treatise that Boyle calls "On Atoms" in his "Materialls & Addenda" of 25 January 1649/50, Boyle praised Gassendi, along with Kenelm Digby and René Descartes, for resurrecting atomistic ideas.[80] Despite this praise, the traditional atheistic stigma attached to atomism made Boyle wary of becoming publicly associated with such ideas, as is evident in the note attached to this draft, which reads: "These Papers are without fayle to be burn't." The ideas that were to form the basis for Boyle's corpuscular philosophy—which attributed operations of nature to the motions of material particles and their consequent organization—were in nascent development at this time. Boyle was not alone in his interest in such interpretations of nature, for the ideas of the French mechanists were being rapidly disseminated in England in this period.[81]

For Boyle, mechanistic hypotheses provided a more fundamental and more logically consistent explanation of natural phenomena than did the arguments from "spiritual principles" and "occult essences" favored by the iatrochemists. Yet predictably, Boyle's focus was not to overthrow iatrochemical ideas with atomistic ones but to unite them. His contemporaries were well aware of this intention, as can be seen in a letter from Robert Southwell to Henry Oldenburg of 1 March 1660, which states, "I am extreame glad to understand that Mr. Boyle is ingaged in soe advantageous a designe as ye collation of Chymicall experiments with Atomicall notions."[82]

Boyle would have been particularly interested in Highmore's atomistic interpretations of both embryological development and "cures by sympathy." He had acquired an interest in the sympathetic cure of wounds quite early, for in the same 25 January 1649/50 list of treatises begun or completed by him in which he refers to the treatise "On Atoms," he lists another entitled "Of the Weapon-salve and occult Qualitys."[83] The treatise is lost, and its specific content unknown. However, we do know that during this time a number of treatises were written about this particular cure. Some were authored by those adhering to the traditional explanation of Paracelsus, who claimed to have discovered this remedy. Paracelsus's view was that the cure of wounds at a distance by use of the "weapon salve" or "powder of sympathy" was explicable in terms of hidden occult sympathies or astral influences. However, a wholly mechanistic interpretation had been provided by Kenelm Digby in 1644, and Boyle may have been aware of this work, since he appears to have been familiar with Digby's atomistic views generally.[84] Since Boyle not only was writing on atomism at this time but also listed as planned or completed a treatise entitled "Of the Effluvia and Pores of Bodys,"[85] it is possible that Boyle too was investigating the possibility of a mechanistic interpretation.

Highmore's "Discourse of the Cure of Wounds by Sympathy" wholly rejected the occult interpretation and maintained that particles of the "weapon salve," when combined with the blood of the victim that was present on the weapon or other object, wafted into the air and were thereby transported to the site of the wound, where they insinuated themselves into pores of the wound naturally suited by size and shape to accommodate them.[86] It is quite possible that Highmore recognized that Boyle would be sympathetic to such an interpretation and that this was one reason prompting him to dedicate *The History of Generation* to Boyle.

The main body of Highmore's text deals with embryology, and here too Highmore may have seen Boyle as both interested in the specific topic and receptive to his interpretation of it. The wording of Highmore's dedication indicates a familiarity with Boyle's experiments and the degree of his skill. Highmore praised Boyle, his "much honoured Friend," as follows: "You have not thought your blood and descent debased, because married to the Arts. You stick not to trace Nature in her most intricate paths, to torture her to a confession; tho with your own sweat and treasure obtained." He ended by saying that he hoped "perhaps something may here be found, that may encourage others to a farther search. *I shall not despair of your own, which may give a better account* and a plenary satisfaction, if it may be, in these so labyrinthean works of Nature."[87] Even allowing for the fact that Highmore might be inclined to flatter Boyle because of his social status, it appears that Highmore had a genuine respect for Boyle's experimental acumen and may have believed in earnest that Boyle was capable of extending knowledge in the area of embryology.

There is evidence that Boyle did engage in embryological investigations for himself. Scattered references to embryological development in his later writings show that he, like Highmore, accepted Harvey's epigenetic views. That he made careful experimental observations of the stages of embryological development is clear from a passage in "Two Essays concerning the Unsuccessfulness of Experiments," published as part of his *Certain Physiological Essays* (1661), in which he mentions that he confronted Highmore with his discovery that there were time discrepancies in the development of different eggs, to which Highmore replied that he too had observed such discrepancies.[88]

Highmore's role in introducing Boyle to the study of human anatomy is indicated in a 1653 letter that Boyle's friend and Highmore's kinsman William Petty wrote to Boyle chiding him for being excessively preoccupied with his own health. Petty suggests: "My cousin Highmore's curious hand hath shewn you so much of the fabric of man's body, that you cannot think but that so complete a piece as yourself will be always at some little fault or other."[89] The proximity of Highmore's home in Shelborne to Stalbridge, added to the fact that Highmore served as physician to Boyle at this time, would have given ample opportunity for Boyle to learn anatomy from Highmore.

In addition to their common interest in atomistic philosophy and anatomical observation, Boyle and Highmore also shared a belief that microscopes were indispensable tools for experimental research. *The History of Generation,* in fact, was the first published work in England to refer to the use of the microscope.[90] Boyle felt the microscope was another means of reading the Book of Nature, as evidenced in a passage from his treatise *Seraphick Love,* completed in 1648 and published in 1659:

> When with excellent microscopes I discern, in otherwise invisible objects, the inimitable subtilty of nature's curious workmanship; and when, in a word, by the help of anatomical knives and the light of chymical furnaces, I study the book of nature and consult the glosses of Aristotle, Epicurus, Paracelsus, Harvey, Helmont, and other learned expositors of that instructive volume: I find myself oftentimes reduced to exclaim with the Psalmist, How manifold are thy works, O Lord? in wisdom hast thou made them all!"[91]

Boyle's belief in the usefulness of microscopes as tools for scientific investigation and not merely as curiosities is also illustrated by a comment made by Hartlib in his *Ephemerides* dated between 8 and 16 January 1651: "Hee (Mr. B.) cares not for optical niceties but as they are subordinate to Natural Philosophy. For by the Microscopes and Tubes that may bee learnt and discerned which cannot bee done neither by Reason or Experiments but only Sense."[92]

Highmore, then, appears to have shared many interests with Boyle and was also in a position to encourage Boyle's investigations of the human body. His work provided Boyle with a perspective on knowledge useful to medicine that differed from the perspective Boyle was then obtaining from his iatrochemist friends in the Hartlibian circle, whose work centered more on pharmacology and therapy.

Boyle's interest in anatomy grew simultaneously with his interest in chemistry, and Hartlib encouraged him in both these pursuits. Boyle traveled to Holland in the spring of 1648, where he probably visited the famed School of Anatomy in Leyden, where he would have observed anatomical dissections, for Hartlib wrote Boyle upon his return, thanking him for his "new discoveries in anatomy."[93]

In part 1 of his *Usefulness of Experimental Natural Philosophy* Boyle speaks of having a fascination with anatomy comparable to that he had with chemistry:

> One should think, Pyrophilus, that the conversing with dead and stinking carcasses (that are not only hideous objects in themselves, but made more ghastly by putting us in mind, that ourselves must be such) should be not only a very melancholy, but a very hated employment. And yet, Pyrophilus, there are anatomists, who dote upon it; and I confess its instructiveness hath not only so reconciled me to it, but so enamored me of it, that I have often spent hours much less delightfully, not only in courts, but even in libraries, than in tracing in those forsaken mansions, the inimitable workmanship of the omniscient Architect.[94]

Later in the same treatise he notes, "And tho my condition does (God be praised) enable me to make experiments by others hands; yet I have not been so nice, as to decline dissecting dogs, wolves, fishes, and even rats and mice, with my own hands."[95]

Highmore was not the only influence upon Boyle in his early exposure to anatomy. Another major contributor to Boyle's early training in that subject was William Petty. Petty (1623–87) had been introduced to Boyle by Hartlib in 1647. Hartlib described Petty as "a most rare and exact anatomist, and excelling in all mathematical and mechanical learning."[96] The earliest known letter from Petty to Boyle, dated 21 June 1648, is a request that Boyle communicate some experiments to him.[97]

At this time Petty was not only interested in anatomical investigation but deeply involved in efforts to reform medical teaching methods by introducing clinical instruction and bedside observation. His first publication, in 1648, entitled *The Advice of W.P. to Mr. Samuel Hartlib,* outlined a proposal for educational reform and contained an elaborate design for a teaching hospital.[98] Petty may have been inspired in his reform efforts by similar attempts then being made to introduce clinical medicine at Leyden and Utrecht. He was well acquainted with these two schools, having spent some time at both when he fled to the Continent upon the outbreak of the English civil war. Petty's proposals for reform of medical teaching fit in well with Hartlib's aims for educational reform as a means to an improved society, and this may well have prompted Boyle's own trip to Holland in 1648.

In 1650 Petty became professor of anatomy at Oxford, where he came to be highly regarded for his prowess in anatomical dissection. (He also gained widespread fame that same year for his involvement in the successful revival of the "executed" criminal Ann Green.)[99] Petty soon became involved in the activities of the Oxford Philosophical Club, which included many of the experimental scientists formerly connected with the London Gresham College Group.[100] (Boyle later was to work with many of these same men after his own move to Oxford in 1655.) The club met for a time at Petty's residence, which was in an apothecary's house and therefore a convenient place for carrying out experiments.

Petty had a particularly good opportunity to guide Boyle's anatomical research when, in late 1651, he was appointed physician-general to the army in Ireland. He arrived in Ireland in 1652, the same year that Boyle traveled to that country for an extended visit on behalf of his family. Boyle remained in Ireland two years. When he wrote Hartlib to complain of his isolation and boredom, due to the lack of laboratory facilities or adequate intellectual contact there, Hartlib suggested that Boyle contact his associates then residing in that country, including Petty. Boyle appears eventually to have taken Hartlib's advice, for in a later letter to Frederick Clodius, Boyle relates that Petty has been assisting him in anatomical investigations:

> For my part, that I may not live wholly useless, or altogether a stranger in the study of nature, since I want glasses and furnaces to make a chemical analysis of inanimate bodies, I am exercising myself in making anatomical dissections of living animals: wherein (being assisted by your father-in-law's ingenious friend Dr. Petty, our general's physician) I have satisfied myself of the circulation of the blood, and the (freshly discovered and hardly discoverable) receptaculum chyli, made by the confluence of the *venae lacteae;* and have seen (especially in the dissection of fishes) more of the variety and contrivances of nature, and the majesty and wisdom of her author, than all the books I ever read in my life could give me convincing notions of. Designing, whilst I am kept prisoner in Ireland, to prosecute that

> study, as I have opportunity; if there be any thing relating to it, wherein my knives may give you any satisfaction, I shall be very proud to employ them to so elevated an end.[101]

Hartlib responded to this news with a request that Boyle keep him informed of Petty's work and with information of his own concerning the latest published work on anatomy in Europe.

Conclusion

It is clear that Boyle acquired a considerable amount of medicine-related knowledge during the period he lived at Stalbridge. He obtained a familiarity with both traditional and chemical medicaments, an understanding of the iatrochemical philosophy, skill in anatomy, and an awareness of the possibility of interpreting organic phenomena and the action of curative agents in atomistic terms. Boyle read widely during this period on many subjects, including medicine, and was kept abreast of the latest medical trends and discoveries by Hartlib. His own preoccupation with his health was both a spur to medical investigation and a psychological hazard. In an April 1653 letter Petty chided Boyle for his hypochondria. While he noted that "this distemper is incident to all that begin the study of diseases," he added that "it is possible, that it hangs yet upon you, according to the opinion you may have of yourself, rather than according to the knowledge that others have of your greater maturity in the faculty." Petty also faulted Boyle for "practising upon yourself with medicaments (though specifics) not sufficiently tried by those that administer or advise them."[102]

Boyle's genuine curiosity about medical matters, coupled with the wariness he had developed in his youth of traditional physick, ensured his keeping an open mind regarding new treatments and remedies. He compiled a considerable amount of information, began setting down his thoughts concerning how to augment medical knowledge, and acquired both experimental and observational skill during his formative years. Boyle's personal ethics led him to the view that investigations of medical subjects, both manual efforts and theoretical speculations, constituted a proper activity for Christian gentlemen, both laymen and medical professionals.

By giving legitimacy to manual activity, Boyle hoped to unite the university-trained physicians, whose expertise was based on book learning and logical analysis, and other classes of practitioners (apothecaries, surgeons, empirics), as well as laymen, in efforts to improve the medical art. This would make the collaborative endeavor more efficient and would encourage better dialogue.

"Divulging of Useful Truths in Physick"

There was a religious dimension to this broad-based investigative activity as well. By laboring together, reading the Book of Nature both to venerate God and to discover and utilize God's gifts to humankind, people could put aside the differences dividing them. Their efforts would lead to the improvement of health and the alleviation of social disorder.

This vision of cooperative work for the betterment of society, which was carefully formulated by Boyle during the difficult years for England which he suffered through while at Stalbridge, was the one he chose to promote and to personally live by. It is the key to understanding the lifelong choices he made concerning his own specific scientific research (particularly those related to medicine) and his choices about whom to associate with and where to reside.

One of these important choices Boyle made in 1655, when he relocated from Stalbridge to Oxford, where he was to live until April 1668. There are several probable reasons for his decision to move there. Many key experimental investigators were emigrating to Oxford at this time, and the creative intellectual environment there was well suited to Boyle's developing scientific interests. The majority of Oxford investigators were physicians or had substantial facility in medicine, and Boyle's own medical interests might have led him there.[103] Boyle had already met John Wilkins (possibly at the instigation of William Petty) in 1653 and thus was aware of the intellectual climate at Oxford and the specific work being accomplished. For Wilkins and others, as for Boyle, science was a means for men of different persuasions to collaborate on neutral ground.

A move to Oxford also may have seemed feasible to Boyle because of the fragmentation in the ranks of the Hartlib circle by this time. Some of the men Hartlib had most trusted to implement his various projects for reform had either left the group or become unreliable (e.g., Worsley, George Starkey, and eventually even Clodius). Others became engaged in petty squabbling, self-absorbed mysticism, or the quest for personal financial gain. Hartlib's grandiose plans had always been predicated upon his acquiring substantial government funding, and this, unhappily, was not forthcoming. During the mid-1650s many iatrochemists in his circle became vocal proponents of the movement to abolish Galenism and base medicine entirely on the philosophies of Paracelsus and Van Helmont. Boyle not only would have deplored such fractiousness but would have rejected the occult explanations of chemical phenomena that permeated iatrochemical theory and led to alliances between chemists holding these views and the radical sectaries.

In assessing the impact of latitudinarian views on scientific development in this period, James and Margaret Jacob suggest that in the 1650s many scientific investigators of moderate outlook "consciously distanced themselves from the radicals who saw in science a powerful tool for promoting religious, political, and social revolution" and retreated to Oxford, where they "pursue[d] their thoughts in quiet contemplation" and developed a matter theory that embodied a "conservative interpretation of the social hierarchy."[104] It is possible that Boyle was influenced in this way to accompany his fellow moderates to Oxford.

Since Boyle left no correspondence in which he revealed his specific reasons for moving to Oxford in 1656, one cannot be absolutely sure of his motives. It is clear, however, that at the time, Boyle felt that he would be welcome there and believed it to be a congenial and intellectually stimulating environment in which to further his scientific work.

The excitement Boyle felt about Oxford science at this time can be sensed from a letter he wrote to Hartlib on 14 September 1655, shortly before taking up residence in Oxford. Boyle reports that he had visited two days with John Wilkins and relates:

> That which most endeared to me my Entertainment was the Delight I had to find there a Knot of such Ingenious and free Philosophers, who I can assure you do not only admit and entertaine Reall Learning, but cherish and improve It, and have done & are like to doe more toward the Advancement of it than any of those Pretenders that doe more busie the Presse and presume to undervalue them, & during the little time I spent there I had the satisfaction to heare both the Chiefe Professors & Heads of Colleges maintain Discourses and Arguments in a way so far from Servile that if all the New Paradoxes have not found Patrons there, tis not their dissent from the Ancient or the Vulgar Opinions but some juster Cause that hinders their admission.[105]

Oxford represents a new phase of Boyle's intellectual development. But this by no means should be construed as a deliberate separation from Hartlib himself or support of projects for social welfare. The tenor of the works Boyle was soon to publish shows that his belief that scientific discovery was useful to society and pleasing to God was as strong as ever. Nor were these ideas foreign to the Oxford scientists as a group. Wilkins and others had a deep concern for these same things.

Boyle's communication with Hartlib did not cease when he moved to Oxford. His contact with Hartlib, in fact, remained regular, as entries in Hartlib's *Ephemerides* show. Boyle continued to support efforts to advance Hartlib's schemes.[106] Nor did Boyle abandon his enthusiasm for at least the more practical ideas of Van Helmont upon moving to Oxford. As Anthony Clericuzio has pointed out recently, "It is evident that at the time of Boyle's move to Oxford, the atmosphere in that city was far from being hostile to iatrochemical ideas, as is shown by Ralph Bathurst's Lectures in 1654 and by Thomas Willis's early work on fermentation and fevers, which circulated in manuscript already in 1656." Clericuzio correctly argues that Boyle's chemical and corpuscular views developed simultaneously throughout this period and that "at the end of the 1650s Boyle shared important aspects of van Helmont's theories and conceived Helmontianism as a radical rupture with the Paracelsian chemical philosophy."[107]

Boyle's scientific interests at Oxford branched out in many directions, yet much of his work still was related to medicine. Building on his background in anatomy and chemistry and on his familiarity with mechanical principles, Boyle directed much of his effort to physiological experimentation, particularly in the areas of respiration and digestion. He also shared his Oxford colleagues' fascination with experiments in blood transfusion. His multifaceted chemical investigations also continued, including considerable work on the action of drugs.

It was during this period that Boyle first began to articulate his basic ideas on matter, nature, and life. A closer examination of these ideas is essential to a full understanding of Boyle's scientific methodology and the philosophical basis of his medical thought.

CHAPTER TWO

Developing a Philosophy of Nature

The Oxford Environment in the Mid-Seventeenth Century

Boyle's move to Oxford brought him into close association with men in the forefront of scientific inquiry of the day. Influenced by Francis Bacon's general schema for advancing knowledge, these men viewed the generation of knowledge as a process by which empirical findings were to be validated not according to how much they agreed with the established theories of traditional authority but by independent confirmation by credible observers.[1] From these men Boyle was to learn firsthand how the study of nature, and particularly of organic phenomena, could be enhanced by concerted, collaborative effort.

Since the organization of the Philosophical Club at Oxford in 1647, quite varied experimental work had been performed there by men such as John Wilkins, Jonathan Goddard, William Petty, and John Wallis. The members of this group may have differed in their religious and political views, as well as in their methodological approaches to scientific investigation, but they all shared a commitment to advancing knowledge beyond that known to the ancients. Removed from the contentious and distracting aspects of life in London, these men found at Oxford a relatively stable and protected environment in which to work.

In September 1653, Wilkins wrote to Boyle encouraging him to come to Oxford, "where you will be a means to quicken and direct us in our enquiries," and noting that he "shall be most ready to provide the best accommodations for you that this place will afford."[2] By the time of this letter, Boyle was already known to many of the men at Oxford. Many of the Oxford investigators communicated freely with Hartlib and his circle. Boyle's close friends Petty and Highmore had worked at Oxford and maintained contacts there. As a result, Boyle was well aware of the scientific work being done there. Boyle probably decided to move to Oxford shortly after receiving Wilkins's letter, for there is evidence that he soon was making preparations to leave Stalbridge. In an October 1653 letter to Boyle, Lady Ranelagh says that she has engaged rooms for him from the apothecary John Crosse, whose house adjoined University College on High Street.[3]

By the time he moved to Oxford, Boyle had developed rather sophisticated experimental skills in chemistry and anatomy and was familiar with the use of scientific tools, such as the microscope. He also had become very conversant in the basic notions of the atomist philosophy, an interest shared by his colleagues Highmore and Petty. While at Stalbridge, Boyle had already become interested in how one might fuse notions of particulate matter and chemical action into a single theoretical framework. His new Oxford colleagues shared Boyle's interest in investigating natural phenomena in terms of atomic and chemical ideas. In fact, Oxford in this period was receptive to many new scientific ideas and had substantial resources to support scientific inquiry and scientific publication. Mid-seventeenth-century Oxford was endowed with seven chairs in science and an excellent library. It also had a growing number of students, as well as several new colleges, and was home to an impressive number of publishing booksellers.[4] It is not difficult to see why it had become a haven for learned gentlemen seeking to expand knowledge of nature beyond the received traditions. Intellectually, Boyle was in good company. As Thomas Birch succinctly put it, "Oxford indeed was the only place in England, where at that time Mr. Boyle could have lived with much satisfaction to himself."[5]

The key men Boyle came into contact with at Oxford in 1653 included John Wilkins, then the undisputed leader of the group of investigators at Oxford Thomas Willis, Richard Lower, Ralph Bathurst, Jonathan Goddard, Christopher Wren, John Wallis, and Seth Ward. These individuals were to take the lead in the rapid development of science and technology in the next decades. Collectively they planned and engaged in a variety of original experiments in the areas of physiology and chemistry and pioneered in the use of scientific instruments.

As a group, the Oxford researchers emphasized the importance of conducting scientific activity in an atmosphere of conscious tolerance for the ideas of others and of exercising great caution before developing their experimental findings into elaborate theoretical systems. Some contemporary authors have suggested that their program of collaboration amounts to a deliberate latitudinarian agenda.[6] Others, such as Hunter, suggest that the decision to maintain a demeanor of "neutrality" and tolerance was simply a procedural expedient to allow men who otherwise may have been ideological opponents to carry on collaborative scientific work.[7] In any case, these Oxford men developed a degree of camaraderie and mutual respect that permitted them freely to share and extend each other's ideas.

Boyle, already imbued with irenical ideals, no doubt applauded this approach toward scientific investigation. Oxford afforded Boyle an excellent environment in which to join other investigators in exploring the Book of Nature for the benefit of humanity. Driven by his own sense of purpose, Boyle viewed his role not only as that of a participant in specific scientific investigations but also as that of a promoter of the general value of scientific inquiry. This explains why Boyle spent a considerable amount of time at Oxford both perfecting his experimental techniques and elaborating a comprehensive explanatory framework for the operations of nature.

Boyle began publishing in earnest at Oxford. Some of the works published in this period were begun while Boyle was still at Stalbridge and reflect the development of his views on atomism and chemistry and the utility of natural philosophy. Other publications are detailed accounts of specific experimental work undertaken at Oxford. Works on theological subjects were published as well, revealing Boyle's continued, consistent interest in religious writing, often with an eye to bridging his scientific outlook and his theological beliefs.[8]

Boyle's reputation as a scientific researcher and theorist was made during his Oxford years. When John Wilkins left in 1659 for Cambridge, Boyle's lodgings became the meeting place for the Oxford virtuosi. There both his Oxford colleagues and a steady stream of visitors could discuss a variety of ideas and test new discoveries.

The Restoration of Charles II in 1660 altered both the scientific and the academic climate in England. Oxford was no longer needed as a refuge by those who had fled London because of their political views during the Protectorate. Charles II wished to be recognized as a patron of science and thus supported the establishment in London of the Royal Society in 1660. This drew a great number of virtuosi to London. Boyle, although a founding member and active participant in the Royal Society, chose to continue to reside in Oxford.

Now both respected in the scientific community and in official favor at the royal court, Boyle was offered many honors, including a peerage, which he refused. Several offices of personal importance to him he accepted, however, including the governorship of the Corporation for Propagating the Gospel in New England and a directorship in the East

India Company. In 1664 he became a member of the Company of Royal Mines. True to his philosophy of creating an improved and more pious society, he utilized these positions to facilitate missionary activities and to encourage scientific inquiry.

During the plague year 1665–66, Boyle relocated to a village several miles from Oxford, taking the opportunity of the privacy this move afforded to consolidate his many notes and manuscript fragments. Only in 1668 did he finally leave Oxford for good. Eventually he took up residence with his sister, Lady Ranelagh, at her London home in Pall Mall. In 1670 he suffered a paralytic stroke. From this time on, he remained in failing health, yet continued his scientific work with the help of his laboratory assistants. Boyle's biographer, Louis Trenchard More, has noted, in fact, that "some of [Boyle's] most important work appeared during the five years following his paralysis."[9] Boyle continued to reside in London until his death in 1691.

Developing an Agenda and a Conceptual Scheme for Science and Medicine

During his residence at Oxford, Boyle developed his general philosophy of nature and a procedural methodology for reforming both science and medicine. In 1663 he published his treatise *Usefulness of Experimental Natural Philosophy,* which he had begun writing at Stalbridge. In this work he presents what amounts to an overall agenda for the study of nature, with the improvement of medicine as a primary target. Part 1 of this work focuses on the advantages of the study of natural philosophy to the general augmentation of knowledge. Part 2 focuses specifically on the utility of natural philosophy to the main categories of learned medicine: physiology, pathology, semiotics, hygiene, and therapeutics.

To support his contention that medicine would benefit from having the widest possible knowledge base, Boyle took great care to enumerate the ways natural philosophers had already furthered medical progress or could do so in the future. He encouraged physicians to consider findings of chemists, anatomists, and empiricists; to conduct their own tests to evaluate the utility of this information; and where appropriate, to incorporate new cures and techniques into their medical practice, regardless of their source. He insisted that physicians, like other researchers, could benefit from the use of any tools that might extend sense perception or help obtain quantitative information.

In short, Boyle championed the idea that an empirical approach, using tools designed to enhance visual perceptions, coupled with a knowledge of chemistry and aided by a rational conceptual framework, afforded the best hope of improving the medical art. This broad-based, collaborative approach would free medical methodology from its overreliance on the written word and traditional authority while preserving medicine from the factionalism of those who sought to overthrow traditional Galenic medicine.

The main thrust of Boyle's treatise is that through collaborative efforts and organized experiment phenomena could be understood in material terms, without recourse to occult explanations. If scientific activity was to be encouraged as a public venture, then the explanatory system had to be one amenable to empirical confirmation and rational analysis. To provide a framework for the rational, wholly physical analysis of nature he preferred, Boyle forwarded what he termed the "corpuscular hypothesis."

The scope of Boyle's operational agenda is perhaps best reflected in a very unpolished poetic sketch that he (or one of his amanuenses) entered into one of his notebooks, now held in the Royal Society. Obviously a rough draft, the poem provides some insight into how Boyle viewed his personal scientific work:

> Th' first sorts of things fit for what I write
> The next do's to Philosophy give much Light
> The third's of things, that few are like to try
> For want of money, skill or Industry
> Th' fourth things of great use to mankind shows
> Easy and cheap, the fifth and last compose.
> The fourth, foretells the Event of untry'd things.
> The 5th the use of apply'd Rations brings.
> The 6th of things whose practice hints doth give
> That from their Bulk and Shape men may derive.
> The 7th their various circumstances shows
> As measure lasting weight, and such as those.[10]

This fragment reveals Boyle's dual concern (1) to extend useful knowledge, particularly in areas that others might not have the facility or resources to investigate, with special attention to discoveries of products that were cheaply and easily prepared, and (2) to provide a rational explanation of phenomena, both in basic atomistic terms (involving "Bulk and Shape") and in more specific, empirical terms ("measure" and "lasting weight"), which give insight into individual qualities of substances.

What is clear from this fragment, other than that Boyle was no poet, is Boyle's belief that nature could be better understood and that useful discoveries could be made by means of a broad-based investigative program.

"Divulging of Useful Truths in Physick"

The Baconian dual emphasis on experiments of light and experiments of fruit is reiterated here. There is a definite belief that valid knowledge of nature is obtainable through human effort.

Although Boyle is commonly recognized for his empiricism, his suggestion that observation might provide "hints" about the "Bulk" and "Shape" of the underlying structure reveals that he was not opposed to formulating hypotheses. The formation of hypotheses was necessary particularly because Boyle rejected the idea that chosen individuals are granted sudden and complete insight into nature by divine illumination. The quest for knowledge of nature Boyle envisioned as being a long-term effort that the investigator engaged in with diligence and patience as an act both of veneration and of charity to improve the human condition. Boyle's rejection of the notion of sudden illumination by divine fiat was only partly due to his opposition to religious enthusiasm. Boyle also suggests that God encourages human beings to apply their own reasoning powers to understanding nature's design because it provides them a good lesson in humility. In the act of searching for knowledge, the individual gains an appreciation not only of the grand and complex design of creation but also of how limited human powers are compared with those of God. While these human investigators can take comfort in the belief that their search is pleasing to God and that their efforts may result in limited discovery, they also become aware that their very humanity flaws their search and permits them, at best, to obtain only a partial understanding of the Design of nature.

The researchers come to recognize that they should treat any information they obtain as incomplete and any analysis based on this information as provisional. Future "discoveries" could necessitate discarding or altering old theories. It was clear, however, that no grand system of nature should be built upon any given set of existing hypotheses, since this would be akin to building upon a foundation of shifting sand. Boyle insisted that the most one could aim for was a set of internally consistent provisional hypotheses. These could serve as a framework for directing further study of natural phenomena. Over time, some hypotheses would prove more comprehensive and more accurate than others. Like Bacon, Boyle saw that a body of knowledge could be built up gradually through continued research and observation, through human effort rather than divine illumination. The formation and validation of hypotheses became the cornerstones of his methodology.

Boyle pointed out both the heuristic purpose and the limitations of hypothesis. He was careful to distinguish the varying levels of comprehensiveness characterizing different hypotheses. These levels are best articulated in a fragment of an unfinished treatise entitled "The Requisites of a Good Hypothesis":

> The Requisites of a good Hypothesis are:
> That it be Intelligible.
> That it neither Assume nor Suppose anything Impossible, unintelligible, or demonstrably False.
> That it be consistent with itself.
> That it be fit and sufficient to Explicate the *Phaenomena,* especially the chief.
> That it be, at least, consistent, with the rest of the *Phaenomena* it particularly relates to, and do not contradict any other known *Phaenomena* of nature, or manifest Physical Truth.
> The Qualities and Conditions of an *Excellent Hypothesis* are:
> That it be not Precarious, but have sufficient Grounds in the nature of the Thing itself or at least be well recommended by some Auxiliary Proofs.
> That it be the Simplest of all the good ones we are able to frame, at least containing nothing that is superfluous or Impertinent.
> That it be the *only* Hypothesis that can Explicate the Phaenomena; or at least, that do's Explicate them so well.
> That it enable a skilful Naturalist to foretell future Phaenomena by their Congruity or Incongruity to it; and especially the events of such Experim'ts as are aptly devis'd to examine it, as Things that ought, or ought not, to be consequent to it.[11]

What is interesting here is that Boyle maintains that *two* main types of hypotheses exist and that both are useful. The "good" hypothesis ties together facts without contradiction and thus is helpful in organizing information. The "excellent" hypothesis, however, goes further; it is, so to speak, the ideal refinement of the good hypothesis, since it provides the *one* most reasonable explanation of the facts as presently known and has the further capability of predicting yet unexamined events.[12] Experiment is the means of confirming hypotheses of *either* type.

Although Boyle took the position that the ultimate secrets of nature could be known fully only to God and that the best an individual could hope to attain was tentative and probabilistic knowledge, he was no pure skeptic. As noted in chapter 1, Boyle maintained that God consistently aided people in their efforts to know nature. This was his way of rewarding the faithful who revered his creation. While he rejected divine illumination as the means by which God augmented human knowledge, Boyle maintained that God aided individuals by protecting their experimental efforts from "those unlucky accidents, which often make ingenious and industrious endeavors miscarry," or by making investigators "dear and acceptable to the possessors of secrets," who can enlighten them concerning knowledge that it would take "many a year's toil and study" to acquire independently. What was most important, God aided investigators' inquiries by "directing them to happy and pregnant hints, which an ordinary skill and industry may so improve, as to do such things, and make such discoveries by virtue of them, as both others, and the person himself . . . would scarce have imagined to be possible."[13]

All this was done in what Boyle would call the usual concourse of nature. No divine intervention was needed. Humanity's acquisition of knowledge was a preordained goal that God actualized without contravening or interrupting the normal course of events. No single individuals were selected to receive truth by divine fiat. The task of advancing knowledge was one best served by cooperative labor. God participated in this process much as a father would guide and encourage the efforts of his children.

Although God might lead people in the right direction, they needed to know when they had discovered something significant. Boyle therefore maintained that at Creation, God had endowed the human rational faculty with an "internal light" by which it could determine the truth or falsity of principles.[14] When a person is brought, through the normal course of investigation, to a position where new discovery is possible, it is the human being that takes the final step to comprehension, aided, however, by means of his or her God-given "internal light" of reason. Boyle's views here appear similar to the Hermetic notion of "right reason," the reasoning faculty improved by divine illumination. That such Hermetic language was indeed widely utilized by seventeenth-century natural philosophers has been discussed at length by Lotte Mulligan.[15] Here Boyle uses the concept to allow for the role of God in the normal course of the generation of knowledge while avoiding acceptance of the idea of sudden illumination of select individuals by divine fiat, an idea that had come to be associated with religious radicalism and dogmatism.

To aid investigators in sorting out the knowledge they had obtained, Boyle distinguished two categories of "truths." On the one hand, "truths" are "complete," "absolute," or "eternal." These are limited to "those theoretical principles and axioms which are the foundations of our reasonings, such as . . . 'two contradictories cannot both be true,' and 'every thing is, or is not.'" "Truths" at this level form the basis for the logical order according to which one is able to make any statements whatsoever concerning the world in which one lives. Other "truths," however, are "gradual";

they are as complete as we can determine, given the present state of our knowledge, but at best they can provide only an partial picture of how things really are.[16]

Boyle especially criticized those mechanists who, although they shared many of his hypotheses about nature, went too far in asserting that their interpretations were "the true and genuine cause of the things they attempt to explicate." Boyle explained that

> as an artificer can set all the wheels of a clock a going, as well with springs as with weights . . . so the same effects may be as well produced by divers causes different from one another; and it will oftentimes be very difficult if not impossible, for our dim reasons to discern surely, which of these several ways . . . he has really made use of to exhibit them . . . and that it is a very easy mistake for men to conclude, that because an effect may be produced by such determinate causes, it must be so or actually is so.[17]

The legacy of humanity's Fall from grace was that one could obtain only imperfect knowledge. One's best efforts would afford only an approximation of how the world worked. Nonetheless, over time, through the united efforts of those who sought to understand nature, better and better approximations could be made concerning how nature operated.

Given this viewpoint, it is clear why Boyle was so concerned to distinguish between a "good" and an "excellent" hypothesis. He needed, and found in "good" hypotheses, a conceptual category for "probationary truths," those truths that were limited but had the potential of fitting into a larger picture. They served as a halfway house on the way to understanding. They provided investigators a sense of achievement, however partial, and could serve as a foundation for additional scientific investigation. Boyle made this very clear in the "Proemial Essay" to *Certain Physiological Essays,* published in 1661:

> I consider . . . that generally speaking, to render a reason of an effect or phaenomenon, is to deduce it from something else in nature more known than itself; and that consequently there may be divers kinds of degrees of explication of the same thing. For although such explications be the most satisfactory to the understanding, wherein it is shewn how the effect is produced by their more primitive and catholick affections of matter, namely, bulk, shape and motion; yet are not these explications to be despised, wherein particular effects are deduced from the more obvious and familiar qualities or states of bodies, such as heat, cold, weight, fluidity, hardness, fermentation, &c. though these themselves do probably depend upon those three universal ones formerly named. For in the search after natural

causes, every new measure of discovery does both instruct and gratify the understanding; though I readily confess, that the nearer the discovered causes are to those, that are highest in the scale or series of causes, the more is the intellect both gratified and instructed.[18]

For "everyday" practical scientific work, the "good" hypothesis held an important place. Boyle's method involved performing experiments, observing the visible effects, obtaining consensus from the community of investigators about what was observed (thus establishing "matters of fact"), and then deriving a series of "good" hypotheses that would provide plausible explanations for the phenomena. There was no requirement that explanations be couched in strictly mechanical terms. In fact, the most useful ones often were those articulated in qualitative, chemical terms. These would suffice to spur the scientific imagination and thus give rise to additional investigations. Even though limited in scope and affording a probable (not certain) interpretation of nature, these explanations could stand on their own and be appreciated as valuable to the processes of knowledge gathering and analysis of experiments. Boyle even went so far as to maintain, in fact, that "the most useful notions we have, both in Physics, mechanicks, Chymistry, & ye medicinal art, are not derivd from ye first principles, but from intermediate Theorys, notions and rules."[19]

Nonetheless, the ultimate goal in understanding nature was to establish hypotheses of the "excellent" type. In Boyle's view, these higher-level hypotheses were not mere conveniences for ordering information; rather, their precepts were more justified (in his phrase, "not Precarious"). Although they provided explanations that were still probable rather than certain, the fact that they *could* be established gave the investigators a goal toward which to aim. The "excellent" hypothesis was broader in scope and could explain a wide variety of natural phenomena. It was valuable in that it offered greater insight into the general workings of nature. The most significant feature of an "excellent" hypothesis was that it had predictive value; it could provide a set of fundamental assumptions that could be used in ordering phenomena and in suggesting interrelations in nature. In sum, it allowed the investigator to reason about the underlying order of things.[20]

Boyle is careful to insist that the postulation of an "excellent" hypothesis does not prevent one from continuing to generate less comprehensive (and therefore lower-level) hypotheses of the "good" type. Both activities take place in tandem. The connection between the two types of hypotheses is that one informs the other. There is no formal requirement that the former be deducible from the latter.

Developing a Philosophy of Nature

For Boyle, the "corpuscular hypothesis" (described below) merited the designation "excellent." It provided the simplest and best available explanation for a wide variety of phenomena, given the present level of human understanding. Boyle spent much of his life showing how the corpuscular hypothesis fulfilled the criteria of the excellent hypothesis.

Boyle hoped to gain support for his corpuscular hypothesis by demonstrating its validity in explaining phenomena on a *case-by-case* basis. As Maurice Mandelbaum noted, "We do not find Boyle putting forward any general methodological postulate that the corpuscular hypothesis would . . . have to apply in all cases whatsoever."[21] To do so would have tended toward system building and an assumption that full certain knowledge was obtainable, concepts that Boyle rejected. Rather, Boyle believed that inferences drawn from comparative observations and experiments would illustrate the comprehensiveness and therefore the value of the corpuscular hypothesis. Over time, the universal applicability of a corpuscular view of nature would be more and more appreciated, enhancing its claim to be designated an "excellent" hypothesis.

The experimental demonstrations that Boyle employed to test his hypothesis were drawn primarily from chemistry and the craft traditions. Concerning the latter, Boyle explains that the tradesman, working by artifice in performing such operations as brewing, baking, and so on, "does but bring visible bodies together after a gross manner, and then leaves them to act one upon another, according to their respective natures. . . . [The] phaenomena of trades . . . shew us nature in motion, and that too, when she is (as it were) put out of her course, by the strength or skill of man, which [is] the most instructive condition, wherein we can behold her."[22] As for chemistry, Boyle tells us that

> there are scarce any experiments, that may better accommodate the [corpuscular philosophy] than those, that may be borrowed from the laboratories of chymists. For first, chymistry enabling us to depurate bodies, and in some measure to analyze them, and take asunder their heterogeneous parts, in many chymical experiments we may better than in others know what manner of bodies we employ, art having made them more simple or uncompounded, than nature alone is wont to present them us. . . . And lastly, the bodies employed by the chymists being for the most part active ones, the progress of nature in an experiment, and the series of successive alterations, through which the matter passes from first to last, is wont to be made more nimbly, and consequently becomes the more easy to be taken notice of and comprehended.[23]

"Divulging of Useful Truths in Physick"

Once the experiments were done and the effects observed, Boyle had to show that a corpuscular explanation could be employed to explain the effects. To do this, since action at the corpuscular level was not directly perceivable by the senses, Boyle resorted to *analogy.* He first assumed that his corpuscles obeyed the same laws of mechanical action as did matter that was perceptible by the senses.[24] He then developed plausible mental pictures of submacroscopic mechanical actions that he felt could explain specific observed events. By this means, Boyle attempted to show how one could describe all of nature in physical terms, using the basic premises of the corpuscular hypothesis. He was particularly interested in generating explanations of this type for natural phenomena heretofore considered occult. For example, he explained the efficacy of amulets by suggesting that the medical gemstone that they contained slowly gave off effluvial particles (i.e., small, insensible parts of itself), which mixed with the surrounding air and were breathed in or passed into the body through the pores of the skin. Once inside, these particles passed into the circulating blood and were carried to appropriate parts of the body, where they performed their specific medicinal actions.[25] That a body could emit effluvial particles is itself suggested by analogy with what was observed in the action of evaporation (for liquid bodies) and in the perception of the presence of odoriferous substances (e.g., cinnamon, camphor). That these particles could be carried by the blood is posited by analogy with what is known of particles in suspension in liquids.

The strength of Boyle's explanations largely depended on the "fit" of the analogies employed. His method required the observer to establish for each event under investigation the analogy that was *most* appropriate. If the analogical argument was persuasive, the explanation was deemed plausible. However crude this approach may seem, the fact remains that direct demonstration was not possible in the corpuscular realm. Analogy thus performed a useful function as a conceptual tool.

By accumulating instances of events that could be explained in terms of corpuscular interaction, Boyle hoped to illustrate that the corpuscular hypothesis was the most preferable of all hypotheses dealing with the nature of matter. But he insisted that one could go no further. He felt that any attempt to build a system upon tentative knowledge, no matter how plausible that knowledge seemed, was pretentious and led to the postulation of unsupportable (and untestable) abstractions. Boyle felt that too facile system building hampered scientific inquiry:

> It has long seemed to me none of the least impediments of the real advancement of true natural philosophy, that men have been so forward to

write systems of it, and have thought themselves obliged either to be altogether silent or not to write less than an entire body of physiology: for, from hence seem to have ensued not a few inconveniences, . . . the worst inconvenience of all . . . is, That whilst this vanity of thinking men obliged to write either systems or nothing is in request, many excellent notions or experiments are, by sober and modest men, suppressed; because such persons being forbidden by their judgment and integrity to teach more than they understand, or assert more than they can prove, are likewise forbidden by custom to publish their thoughts and observations, unless they were numerous enough to swell into a system.[26]

System building was also associated with the sin of pride or excessive dogmatism. It was contrary to that charity toward others (including a charitable attitude toward others' viewpoints) that was for Boyle a necessary moral imperative for the Christian gentleman. It led people to hold opposing opinions, thus fragmenting the quest for knowledge and also frustrating the attempt to improve society and achieve religious unity through collaborative effort. Boyle's negative attitude toward system building has its basis, then, more in religious ethics than, as might be imagined, in philosophical skepticism.[27] John Henry has noted that it was important for experimental philosophers to deny certainty in their explanations of natural phenomena lest their philosophies be commandeered by sectarian radicals as "undeniable support" for their world-views.[28] Boyle would have been sensitive to this danger.

Because Boyle always maintained that his corpuscular views had the status of hypothesis, not truth, he ensured that scientific knowledge was to be driven by facts, not theory. He insisted that even those observations and experimental findings that could not easily be fit into any current hypothesis should be collected and evaluated. These anomalous bits of information would in time be explained as the effort to perfect causal hypotheses continued and as God chose to reveal a bit more of his design to human investigators.

The Corpuscular Hypothesis

During his first years at Oxford Boyle spent much time refining this corpuscular view of nature, borrowing extensively from earlier writers, yet adding some embellishments of his own and in particular using his knowledge of chemistry to enhance his more strictly mechanical views. As noted in chapter 1, Boyle had become familiar with the essential ideas of the atomistic philosophy, particularly as expounded by the French philosopher and Catholic priest Pierre Gassendi, at quite an early age.[29] Gassendi held that atoms, initially put in motion by God at the Creation, combined to form "moleculae" (Boyle was to use the term "corpuscle"), which differed according to shape, size, and motion. These concretions gave rise to the observed qualities of objects in nature. In contrast to Descartes', Gassendi's model of nature was more structural than kinetic. Qualitative change in nature was explained in terms of effluvial activity (effluvia being submacroscopic exhalations of a specific qualitative nature and chemical content that sloughed off from gross bodies). Nathaniel Highmore, as has been seen, also used effluvial action in his explanation of the sympathetic action of the "weapon salve." Boyle was to center much of his medical explanation on this concept of effluvial action, using it to describe the spread of contagious disease, the action of disease entities within the human body, and the chemical operations of specific drugs.

One of the clearest summaries of just what the corpuscular hypothesis entailed is provided in "History of Particular Qualities," prefixed to his *Tracts about the Cosmical Qualities of Things,* which was published in 1671. Boyle here posited the principles that illustrated that "the . . . catholick affections of matter are manifestly deducible from local motion; and . . . that these principles being variously associated, are so fruitful, that a vast number of qualities and other phaenomena of nature may result from them."[30] The similarities between Boyle's views of nature at its most basic level and those of Gassendi are considerable.

The first four of the principles Boyle puts forth are, for him, the primary ones:

1. Because "local motion belonging to some parts of the universal matter does not at all tend the same way, but has various determinations in several parts of that matter," it follows that matter is divided into finite parts.
2. Each of these divisions has some defined "bigness or size."
3. Each division also has some determinate shape.
4. Although matter as a whole is in motion, not all parts of universal matter are in motion at any given time, since some motions mutually impede the motion of some parts, or a part may transfer its motion to other bodies. Such parts are in a state of rest. Therefore, the two basic states of matter are "in motion" and "at rest." (It should be noted that this is an inertial concept.)[31]

These finite parts of matter produced by local motion are themselves made up of smaller, insensible particles called "corpuscles," and it is the differentiation at this level that is perceived as the variety of qualities of objects. The remaining principles describe matter at this corpuscular level:

5. All corpuscles have a distinctive "posture or position" with respect to other bodies.
6. All corpuscles are perceived to have an "order or consecution," which allows us to say that "one is before or behind another."
7. All corpuscles associated together in one mass or body have a distinctive "texture" that differentiates them from other associations.
8. Because of the irregularity and difference of the figures of bodies, very few bodies can touch one another so as to leave no intervals between them. Therefore, almost all solid bodies "and those fluid ones that are made up of grosser parts" have pores.
9. Some particles adhere to the aggregate so loosely or are so small that agitation (by heat and other agents) causes them to separate off from the bodies to which they belong. These emissions are called "effluviums."
10. There are three types of aggregations of corpuscles: (*a*) "primary concretions or elements of things," which are durable and uneasily dissoluble clusters of particles; (*b*) "compounded bodies," created by the mingling of primary concretions; and (*c*) "decompounded bodies," created by the mingling of compounds.
11. Every distinct portion of matter (whether corpuscle, primary concretion, or mixture) is to be considered not *in vacuo* but in the context of the whole of nature (i.e., in terms of how it is governed by the "universal fabrick of things" and the "laws of motion established by the author of nature in the world").

These basic principles of the corpuscular hypothesis allowed Boyle to subsume a great number of empirical observations under a single explanatory umbrella. To his mind, the advantage of this explanatory framework was its comprehensiveness and its ability to provide a simple interpretation of the dynamic activity in nature, without need of postulating occult forces, vital spirits, or innate appetites. Boyle felt that phenomena heretofore explained in Aristotelian or Helmontian terms now could be reinterpreted in corpuscular terms.

Although his earliest work on atomism, including the fragment "Of ye Atomicall Philosophy," written between 1651 and 1653, and the first essays of *Usefulness of Experimental Natural Philosophy,* show some sympathy with traditional Epicurean views, Boyle soon after took pains to portray his corpuscular theory of matter as not Epicurean.[32] Boyle's preoccupation with distinguishing his views from Epicurean atomism stemmed partly from his wish to avoid the charge of atheism but also from his desire to broaden the theoretical base to include more qualitative (and chemical) considerations of the behavior of matter.

Boyle carefully developed a classification of corpuscles.[33] Clericuzio has discussed how this classification is essential in providing a theoretical basis for his chemical studies.[34] At the most basic level were *minima naturalia.* Although Boyle initially had written of minima as having chemical properties (in his early treatise fragment "Of ye Atomicall Philosophy"), he now visualized them as wholly mechanical, leaving chemical distinctiveness for second-order corpuscles in his classificatory system. Nonetheless, Boyle still maintained that at this most basic level, one could not assume that the *minima naturalia* were ultimate, indivisible particles, for to require indivisibility would limit the omnipotence of God. For the cautious, nondogmatic Boyle, all that one could say was that *minima naturalia* were insensible particles of matter, each of which "though it be mentally, and by divine Omnipotence divisible, yet by reason of its smallness and solidity nature doth scarce ever actually divide it."[35]

Second-order corpuscles were *primary* (or "primitive") *concretions,* "made up of the coalition of several of the *minima naturalia.*"[36] Still more complex bodies, aggregates of corpuscles, were *compound bodies* (formed by the union of several types of primary concretions) and *decompounded bodies* (a union of different compound bodies). Corpuscular aggregates above the level of *minima naturalia* were qualitatively distinct. The structural differences between these corpuscular aggregates made them behave in a characteristic manner and also interact with other corpuscles in specific ways. Therefore, matter at this level *could* be investigated chemically. Because of this hierarchical classification, chemistry becomes a valid way of examining the world that is separate from, *yet wholly compatible with,* the mechanical world-view.[37]

In order to fully understand the behavior of matter, one had to consider all types of corpuscles in their natural context. This is essentially a holistic view and one that differs from strict Cartesian reductionism. It also should be noted that Boyle's is a structural view, closer to that of Gassendi than to that of Descartes, who focused his efforts on developing a kinetic model. This last point becomes especially significant when considering Boyle's use of the concept of elasticity to explain the tendency of aggregates of matter to preserve their structural viability.

Boyle held that matter must be acted upon by something external to it in order for a change of state to occur. He maintained that matter itself has no plastic power or sentience. The promulgator of motion is God himself. By 1653 Boyle wholly had rejected the Epicurean idea that motion was essential to matter. His attacks on self-moving atoms are, in Clericuzio's words, "unambiguous."[38] Change in nature occurs either in accordance with the laws of motion God established at the Creation or, more rarely, as a result of direct divine intervention. Most of the time, nature's operations follow the laws of motion God decreed as part of his original design. Knowing this affords man the possibility of generating at least some basic hypotheses on how the world works. But God is not constrained by his established order, nor has he removed himself as a direct participatory agent in nature. Quite the contrary. God diligently watches over his creation and may intervene when he sees fit. This explains, of course, how miracles can occur. This view is consistent with voluntarist theology, which holds that God can do anything by fiat and is not constrained in any way.

Boyle, in fact, faulted both Cartesians and Epicurean atomists for failing to recognize God's direct influence in nature's operations. Although he defended the Cartesian position against the charge of atheism, Boyle castigated Descartes for not having "ascribed to the divine Author of nature a more particular and immediate efficiency and guidance in contriving . . . that great engine we call the world."[39] As Boyle explains, God "has at command so many differing and excellent methods and tools, to accomplish what he designs, and does oftentimes actually employ them, for the preservation and welfare of beasts, and even of plants [and] can never want means to compass his most wise and just ends, in relation to mankind; [he is] able, by ways that we should never dream of, to execute his menaces, and fulfill his promises."[40] God's design, under most circumstances, is carried out according to the established laws of nature, but Boyle wanted to assert clearly that God's power is in no way limited by these laws.[41]

Clearly, such a view of God's overseership avoids the pitfall of the Epicurean atomists, who saw activity in nature as random and blind, leaving no place for God. On the other hand, Boyle avoids a "vitalist" explanation, which endows brute matter with inherent "active principles," which would also diminish God's role. Boyle treads a careful path between these two extremes.

Some recent authors, such as John Henry, have suggested that seventeenth-century English mechanists prior to Newton, including Boyle, actually did endorse the idea of "active principles."[42] Henry reasons that many well-known matter theorists, including Boyle, felt the strictly mechanical conception of matter forwarded by Descartes to be so inadequate that it became common to "superadd" to the concept of matter the notion of active principles, both to evade the atheistic implications of mechanism and to fill a "useful explanatory role." Henry forwards this view as a corrective to the view that the reintroduction of occult qualities into natural philosophy was solely the work of Newton.[43]

Henry maintains that Boyle and other pre-Newtonian matter theorists needed active principles to account for physical phenomena for which there was no strict mechanical explanation. Otherwise the only alternative would be to explain such phenomena in terms of perpetual miracles and God's direct intervention, an unsatisfactory solution, since it compromised the idea that nature was orderly, predictable, and ultimately knowable. However, Clericuzio has challenged Henry's view as it is applied to Boyle, pointing out that Boyle did not posit active principles intrinsic to matter but rather active *corpuscles*.[44] This is a correct analysis and an important distinction, since the notion of active corpuscles retains the consistency of the mechanical hypothesis (keeping motion external to matter) while highlighting the importance of texture, or the overall configuration of corpuscles, in which the design itself determines the motion. The design, of course, is God-created, and therefore God's directive role in the regular operations of nature is secure; there is no need for repeated miraculous intervention.

In Boyle's view, then, matter was not inherently active. Nonetheless, aggregates of corpuscles could exhibit qualitative changes that could be understood through chemical analysis. Boyle's postulation of levels of hypothesis allowed him freely to discuss the qualitative interactions of second-order corpuscles (primary concretions) that were endowed with chemical properties without compromising his basic mechanistic perspective. He was convinced that much important information about the constitution of natural substances would be gained as chemical investigators became more proficient and as better methods of chemical analysis became available. He strongly believed that eventually investigators would discover far more basic chemical constituents of substances than those heretofore discoverable via fire analysis. Yet all would still be referable to the main mechanical principles of the corpuscular philosophy. The advantage Boyle saw in his corpuscular hypothesis was that it was flexible enough to allow ample opportunity for reasoned investigation of the qualitative differences between substances and speculation about the more basic universal principles of nature.

Life as Organization

Boyle hoped that the corpuscular hypothesis, because of its comprehensiveness and the simplicity of its formulations, would not only bring about a better conceptual understanding of natural phenomena in general but shed light on the most complex of earthly phenomena—organic life. "Life" was then, as now, difficult to define and describe. Boyle sought to establish a working definition in wholly physical terms, without relying on occult principles or spiritual essences.

The attempt to derive a physical description of how organic bodies operated immediately brought Boyle to an evaluation of the role of the soul. Boyle's own articulation of how the soul affected the body was not always logically consistent. His efforts to depict life in physical, material terms matched in degree of intensity and sophisticated reasoning the efforts of others who sought at that time to extend mechanical explanations to the realm of the living. Like his Oxford colleagues, who aimed to describe physiological phenomena in atomistic and chemical terms, Boyle blended his knowledge of chemistry with his corpuscular perspective in depicting organic function. This gave a qualitative dimension to his perceptual framework, which allowed him to view the human body in a way significantly different from Descartes' representation of the body-as-machine.

In Boyle's day there was a lack of consensus over just what constituted living things. This was an age in which many believed that minerals "grew" in the earth, so the distinction between the "life" of rocks and the "life" of plants and animals was difficult to express. Boyle fully recognized the great need for a more rigorous definition of the term and publicly called attention to this need in his "Three Considerations about Subordinate Forms," an essay contained in his *Origin of Forms and Qualities.* Here he lamented that not only was there confusion over the term "life" as applied to different realms of being—plants, stones, and even incorporeal beings—but people did not even agree on what constituted *animal* life per se, citing the failure of consensus over "whether prolifical, but as yet unhatched, eggs have life or no" or whether flies in winter, when they are in a state seemingly devoid of sense and motion, are truly dead or only "benumbed."[45]

Boyle's own views on life grew out of his ideas on corpuscular aggregation. He came to perceive life as a special case of motion or activity resulting from a specific corpuscular organization. Thomas Hall has termed this view "emergentist."[46] Although this organization occurs automatically when appropriate corpuscles interact, Boyle's perception is not one of blind mechanism. Just as he had maintained for matter in general, he posits that the resultant organization of matter defined as "life" is part of God's predetermined design of nature. The teleological aspect for Boyle is primary. Certain matter was destined to become organized in such a way as to be named "living"; such organized matter, though essentially no different from matter making up "non-living" objects, could be identified by the characteristic motility arising out of its "textural" configuration.

Boyle took great exception to the scholastic Aristotelian view, also teleological, which held that life was determined by the presence of an intrinsic "specific form" (which held dominion over the body components during life and defined that body as an entity) and an immaterial soul (which was the ultimate activating principle). The specific form supposedly was abolished when the soul left the body at death. However, since it was well known that the body does not immediately disintegrate upon death, but maintains its former appearance, at least for a time, even though the form is gone, an additional category—"subordinate forms"—had to be postulated. These "subordinate forms" were said to be present (in a state of potentiality) in each particular body component during life but were under the domination of the specific form. Only upon death (when the "specific form" ceased to be present) did the "subordinate forms" become manifest to maintain, albeit temporarily, the integrity of these separate components and thus give the appearance that the body's form as a whole remained intact.

Boyle did not admit the reality of substantial forms. In his view, they were occult and provided no possibility of being investigated. Therefore, these scholastic Aristotelian definitions of life and death were unsatisfactory to him. In "Three Considerations about Subordinate Forms," he relegated the terms "specific form" and "subordinate form" to the category of mental conveniences.[47] However conceptually valuable they might seem in allowing us to identify the combination of body components as a distinct entity, they should by no means be considered active agents delimiting or maintaining that organized whole.

Boyle preferred to provide an alternative explanation of body integrity entirely in terms of the corpuscular philosophy. He forwarded the holistic idea that the combined interactions (at the corpuscular level) of the body components themselves produced a whole having distinct characteristics not found in the components considered separately. No superimposed "specific form" was needed, therefore, to establish the integrity of the body: the integrity arises from the structural pattern itself.

As Dudley Shapere has noted, this view owes much to the principle of inertia, whereby matter is considered inert and passive and continues in its present state of rest or motion until acted upon by something external to it.[48] With regard to body integrity, Boyle held that even when "hostile agents or causes" resulted in eliminating life from the body, the outward appearance of organization would be retained "until some competent agent put the body out of that state wherein, upon the form's decease, it was left."[49] Change of state, then, and not maintenance, required an agent. This is an important point, since it freed Boyle from the necessity of postulating an external "mover" maintaining life, permitting him to concentrate on forces altering the status quo.

If Boyle questioned the need for substantial and subordinate forms, he also criticized the scholastic view of the role of the soul. He denied that in death the *only* change was the loss of the animating soul, the body being left completely intact but without mobility:

> For tho it may be true, that the visible fabrick may continue for a while without any manifest alteration, yet who can assure us that the internal organization is not considerably changed and vitiated? For the body of an animal is an engine, that consists not only of solid and stable parts, as bones, muscles, skin, . . . but of divers soft ones, as the brain, nerves, etc. and of some that are fluid, as the blood and other liquors; and, which is in our case exceedingly considerable, requires a convenient coaptation, or composition of all these: whence it follows, that the external frame of the body remaining unaltered, yet upon death there may be great and sad alterations in the texture of the blood and humours, and the contexture or structure of other internal parts. And these changes may quite spoil the organization of the body and make it unfit to perform the wonted functions of such an engine.[50]

Death, then, was to be viewed as a physical alteration of the "texture" or configuration of body components, not just as the removal of the "animating" soul. This alteration takes place at the subvisible (corpuscular) level, thus making it impossible to use gross observation of the physical form of the solid parts of the body to determine the life state—or its lack.

Boyle maintained, furthermore, that many of the body processes for which the soul was said to be the *causa motiva* could not be correlated directly with the soul's presence or absence. For example, he cited several life functions thought to be animated by the soul that continued to occur in corpses where the soul was obviously not present, such as the continued growth of a dead man's nails and the discharge of excrements from dead bodies. Boyle also reminded his readers of various processes that, under certain circumstances (or bodily states), could be suspended even though the soul was still present, as "in sudden palsies, tho there be usually no visible change in the affected limb, yet it loses sense, or motion, or both: and not only in syncopes or great swoonings, and in apoplexies, a great part of the animal functions are for the time suspended or unperformed; but even in so natural a state as sleep, the body appears not to move, nor do sounds and odours affect the senses, as when one is awaked, tho the soul be present in the body, and the ears and nostrils be open." Boyle concluded that "in animals some things that are confidently presumed to be the proper effects of the animal's soul, may be really performed by the texture of the body, and the ordinary and regular concourse of external causes."[51]

Boyle sometimes spoke of the soul in materialistic terms. Thomas S. Hall concludes that "Boyle's intention was both to dispense with soul where it seemed unneeded and to give it, where needed, if not actually a physical character, a physical *modus operandi*."[52] This physical dimension, perceived as "directive" activity, was actually referable to corpuscular interactions prompted by the unique configuration of corpuscles in the body. Boyle's aim was to eliminate the need for recourse to an intrinsic spiritual essence to explain ordinary activity, emphasizing that the dynamics of natural phenomena were "built in" to God's original design. No intermediary was required to actuate routine events. (God could directly intervene, of course, and shape particular situations, but he was not constrained to do so; in fact, he superseded the laws of nature—and his design—infrequently.)

Boyle's view assumes that the sum of natural motion will not dissipate, only that the living body, in its physical environment, will be prone to alterations in motion that could compromise its optimal functioning. The reason the living being does not last forever is that nature impinges and motions inevitably are altered, thus changing the "texture" of the organism to one more difficult to maintained.

In the eighteenth century, François Boissier de Sauvages was to qualify this image of the living body. While he shared Boyle's view of the body as a hydraulic engine, Sauvages, whose view was ultimately more quantitative and Newtonian, recognized that the effects of friction and mutual attraction of particles would cause some motion to be lost. Therefore an immaterial source of motion had to be posited; this source he identified with the soul.[53]

Boyle, however, was anxious to eliminate immaterial intermediaries from his discussion of the physical body. To distinguish life from death (or non-life), then, he urged that we try to assess, not whether a spiritual agent is present, but rather whether the overall "textural configuration" (i.e., the combination of structural integrity and dynamic activity) is adequate to sustain the organism. Boyle does not see life and death as substantive opposites; his formulation is more a relativistic continuum leading from life to a number of diseased states to death. The degree of functional capability determines which label we give to each state.

The investigation of how organized matter moves from a healthy state to disease to death is the primary focus of the physician. Since motion is the key to understanding alterations of texture, the physician must concentrate his attention less on the body's solid structures than on the body's fluid parts, and he also must consider the impact of heat and air on the body. The whole focus is on physical agents acting in a physical manner.

In a long passage in "Three Considerations about Subordinate Forms" Boyle provides the analogy of a water mill to illustrate the importance of fluids to maintenance of life. Just as the running water is the source of the motion of the mill, so a plant's sap or juice, "whereof the soul chiefly consists," enlivens the plant. When the source of animation ceases to be present (as would occur in the water mill when the water freezes or in the plant when a rose is plucked from a bush), "nothing that is substantial perishes, but only the particular modification, that resulted from the peculiar kind of union of the more permanent [solid] parts with those congruously shaped and fitly agitated fluid ones, that permeated them."[54] For Boyle, healthy body function is directly dependent upon the continued (and unaltered) flow of body fluids. If the movement of fluids changes to produce a new composite of interactions less advantageous to the efficient operations of the body, disease results. The extreme modification—cessation of fluid flow altogether—is identified as death.

Heat is also a basic consideration, for it is heat that puts the fluid particles (corpuscles) into motion. Boyle's position here was very similar to that of Descartes, who emphasized that the heat of the body, rather than the soul, was the primary cause of physiological activity. The idea of a vital flame requisite to life was hardly new, but during the seventeenth century it received novel mechanistic and chemical interpretations. Heat was directly correlated with motion: the greater the heat, the greater the degree of agitation of the affected particles. A properly maintained vital heat was necessary for health. Too little or too great a heat created modifications perceived as diseased states or, in the extreme, caused death.

Boyle gave much attention to the concept of heat in his works and even devoted an entire treatise to cold, which he treated as a special case of heat. (For Boyle, then, heat and cold were no more absolute opposites than life and death.) Since particles in agitation could reassociate as well as disassociate, Boyle saw heat as having a generative as well as a disintegrative capacity. This point is clearly emphasized in his *Sceptical Chymist,* where much of Boyle's argument against the iatrochemists' assertion of the *tria prima* as the fundamental chemical building blocks of nature was based on the fact that the iatrochemists' had wrongly reached this conclusion when they subjected chemical compounds to fire analysis. According to Boyle, the heating process did not simply reduce substances to their ultimate constituents but may have created new substances by causing recombinations and changes in texture; therefore, the empirical "proof" of the iatrochemist's theories was flawed.[55]

The generative capacity of heat was also important to Boyle's explanations of embryological development and spontaneous generation. He maintained that "no new substance is in generation produced, but only that which was pre-existent obtains a new modification or manner of existence." Heat was necessary to set in motion the constituent particles, which were then to undergo recombination. Boyle's main criticism of those who wished to postulate that a "plastick principle" guides development was that they failed to recognize that this principle "must act after a physical manner."[56] He rejected the idea of a spiritual and immaterial vitalistic force, just as he had rejected other "occult" qualities and the notion of "substantial forms." He insisted that physical effects should have physical efficient causes. Boyle chose to explain spontaneous generation arising from decaying bodies by suggesting "some seminal particles undiscernedly lurking in some part of the destroyed body . . . excited and assisted by a genial and cherishing heat so to act upon the fit and obsequious matter, wherein it was harboured, as to organize and fashion that disposed matter according to the exigencies of its own nature."[57] "Its own nature," of course, was that blueprint built into the original design of creation by God.

The seminal principles Boyle had in mind were a special type of compound corpuscles that had the power of fashioning other particles.[58] These compound corpuscles had been designed by God "with a peculiar texture that was responsible for their power of generating new living beings."[59] In other words, they were programmed in accordance with a divine design. Note that the power of generation is an outgrowth of the "texture," the unique corpuscular configuration, and not a directive principle lodged within matter itself. Here Boyle's logical consistency reveals itself clearly: although he does not attempt to explain generation in strictly mechanical terms, his explanation is not incompatible with the mechanical world-view. Boyle avoids positing any animating powers to brute matter and simply forwards the notion that the generative capacity is a specific type of motion that occurs when certain corpuscular configurations are present—just as God had designed it.

Air was also important to the sustaining of life. The idea of air (with the connotation "divine breath") as a vivifying principle dates back to primitive religion and was maintained by the Stoics. The Aristotelian view, still prevailing in the seventeenth century, saw the function of respiration as cooling the heart, the seat of the vital heat, thus protecting the body against overheating, which would be detrimental to the health of the organism. Galen had pictured the vital heat as fueled by the blood (or some substance contained in the blood), much as a lamp is fueled by oil. As the utilization of oil by the lamp leaves a sooty residue, so in the body sooty wastes are built up. Galen, therefore, added to Aristotle's view of respiration the idea that this sooty waste is removed in exhalation.

Boyle is well known for his work on respiration, particularly experimentation employing the air pump, which challenges and qualifies these earlier ideas. This work is summarized in chapter 3; here it suffices to note that Boyle treated air, not as elemental, but as a heterogeneous body capable of producing effects both as a whole (i.e., via its ability to exert pressure, which he referred to as its "spring") and by virtue of its parts (e.g., via chemical substances carried in it).

Boyle's interest in the "spring" and "elasticity" of the air ultimately led him to formulate the law that bears his name. His attention to pneumatics also led him to suggest how the pressure of the air might affect the human body. Moreover, he sought to articulate a model of the body itself as a "hydraulico-pneumatic engine." His perceptual model of the living body was one of an organized system fed by conduits filled with fluid and airy corpuscles having specific physico-chemical characteristics.

The Human Body as Machine

The conceptualization of the human body as a machine was an important extension of the mechanical philosophy in the seventeenth century. Providing one of the most viable perceptual alternatives to the increasingly challenged Galenic explanations of physiological function in terms of natural faculties, the model of the body-machine held great appeal for those anxious to assimilate the new anatomical discoveries and new forms of localized drug treatment then being advanced into a comprehensive medical philosophy. In addition, the prospect of rendering complex vital operations comprehensible in terms of a simpler mechanics was attractive to many who wished to interpret biological phenomena in materialistic or quantifiable terms.

The use of mechanical models to interpret physiological activity was familiar to the Greeks[60] and is, in fact, a recurring idea in intellectual history, but the visualization of the body as a machine attained special stature in the course of the Scientific Revolution. The ideas of both Descartes and Boyle were influential in articulating this notion.

Descartes' discussion of the body-machine concept predates that of

Boyle by several decades. He devoted several treatises to developing his mechanistic ideas of physiological processes, including his *Treatise on Man,* which was written in the early 1630s but suppressed during his lifetime;[61] his *Discourse on Method,* published in 1637, which contains significant paraphrases from the *Treatise on Man;* and his *Description of the Human Body* (also known as *Formation of the Fetus*), unfinished at his death in 1650 and first published posthumously in 1664. In these works, Descartes explored the extent to which life functions could be explained in wholly mechanical terms, by viewing vital activities as being derived ultimately from the interaction of variously configured, moving particles of matter. Gross anatomy, Descartes believed, revealed important clues regarding these subvisible mechanisms, which were responsible for the growth and maintenance of the organism and its varied observable movements. During the twenty years Descartes spent in Holland (1629–49) he engaged in anatomical dissection, probably using not human cadavers but animal specimens obtained from slaughterhouses. From his observation of structural arrangement and his knowledge of the use of parts, he was able to make inferences about the mechanisms below the level of sense perception that manifested themselves as visible actions of specific organs.[62]

Utilizing his deductive methodology, Descartes tried to account for a wide variety of vital operations, in intricate, if speculative, detail. His aim was to provide a logically consistent picture of life that did not require the postulation of innate faculties or occult causative forces. By careful circumscription of the activities of the rational soul, Descartes was able to forward a strictly mechanical interpretation of all human functions, excepting those related to volition and conscious awareness. By this separation of the physical from the spiritual, he hoped to integrate physiology into the larger superstructure of his physical theory of nature.

To develop his mechanical description of the body, Descartes chose to deal with his subject in idealized terms. Not the human body as it exists in the world, but an "earthen machine" made up of parts totally analogous to those of actual living bodies was the basis for discussion in his *Treatise on Man.* The reasons for employing this idealized model were several. First, Descartes wished to emphasize the conceptual difference between his formally deduced description of body processes and one that simply built upon the erroneous opinions of past scholars. Second, he hoped by this idealization to highlight how fully one could explain body processes in strict mechanical terms—without reference to the soul. Descartes likened his approach to that of a painter who is unable to represent a three-dimensional object upon a two-dimensional canvas and therefore makes a conscious choice to depict in detail one side only of this solid object, leaving the remainder in shadow.[63] Descartes may also have chosen to refer to a strictly idealized model of the body because such a device permitted him to isolate the normative activity of the body from the various and distracting external influences of the natural environment. In his later work *Formation of the Fetus,* Descartes dispensed with the "earthen machine" analogue completely and appeared to address the subject of the body as it is conventionally understood. This was not due to a rejection of the automaton analogy but rather was a response to the need to include contextual considerations in his discussion of generation.[64] However, in his fullest treatment of the body-machine, in the *Treatise on Man,* Descartes' aim clearly is to argue the intelligibility of the body-machine concept, not the reality of the model.

In developing his mechanical description of the body, Descartes relied on several basic assumptions. Primary among these was the idea that nature acts by the "simplest and easiest" means. He also held that the total amount of motion in the universe is constant. The corollary to this requirement—that motion can be transferred from body to body without a change in the total quantity of motion—made possible those cycles of particle displacement and replacement that were so basic to his portrayal of physiological growth and maintenance. Finally, the concept of inertia played an important role in the development of his physiological model, since it allowed him, among other things, to discuss differences in particle speeds on the basis of the degree to which these particles, once set in motion, had been deflected from their original paths. This differential in speed of particles was used to account qualitatively for various vital activities.

Descartes' model of the body-machine served multiple purposes for him. First, it illustrated how successfully one could apply his deductive method to obtain a coherent and comprehensive explanation of even complex natural phenomena. This underscored the value of his methodology. Second, by establishing that life processes could be satisfactorily articulated in mechanistic terms, Descartes was able to argue the essential unity of nature, wherein the same *laws* that applied to physical events in nature at large also pertained to vital function. Particles moved identically whether they were located in the body or in the larger world. Descartes maintained that understanding the body as one understood the operations of the universe as a whole—in terms of a material, dynamic, fully integrated system—was a valuable conceptual stimulus to pragmatic inquiry leading to the improvement of human health.

Unlike Descartes, Boyle wrote no treatises specifically devoted to the concept of the body as a machine. Rather, he appears to have accepted from the outset the general utility of visualizing the body as an "engine" and to have employed mechanical notions where he felt they were appropriate to specific arguments. Thus, Boyle was not seeking to articulate a full-fledged model of the body as a machine but, rather, wished to use the body-machine analogy as a tool to augment understanding of physiological process. Descartes had resorted to speculative but logical reasoning to "flesh out" his model; Boyle rejected such an approach, preferring to hold out the body-machine idea as a fruitful but incomplete framework for experimental research. Additional empirical work might, indeed, allow greater elaboration on the framework and increase the plausibility of the model, but Boyle was not willing to extend himself beyond the evidence available to develop the model itself. Again, underlying this was the idea of avoiding dogmatism.

Like Descartes, Boyle saw the perceptual value of positing mechanisms operative at the subvisible level to explain visible activity in nature. He shared Descartes' belief that a physical model of the body provided a means of increasing our comprehension of physiological events in a way both aesthetic and economical and free from obscure notions, such as "occult principles." The visualization of the body as a finely tuned, fully integrated system, furthermore, seemed to Boyle to provide convincing evidence that the observed world was not the result of chance events, but a product of divine craftsmanship.

Also like Descartes, Boyle focused his attention on the dynamic aspects of his model. Yet there was an important difference. In the most succinct statement of his views on the body as machine, in his treatise *Free Inquiry into the Vulgarly Received Notion of Nature,* published in 1685, Boyle begins with a an emphasis on the human body as a composite of solid, fluid, and spirituous (i.e., gaseous) parts so aggregated as to perform the functions appropriate to the organism. "I look," he wrote, "not on a human body as on a watch or a hand-mill, i.e. as a machine made up only of solid, or at least consistent parts; but as an hydraulical, or rather hydraulopneumatical engine, that consists not only of solid and stable parts, but of fluids, and those in organical motion." So far, this is not inconsistent with Descartes' dynamic model. However, Boyle immediately goes on to add: "And not only so, but I consider, that these fluids, the liquors and spirits, are in a living man so constituted, that in certain circumstances the liquors are disposed to be put into a fermentation or commotion, whereby either some depuration of themselves, or some discharge of hurtful matter by excretion, or both, are produced, so as, for the most part, to conduce to the recovery or welfare of the body."[65] Boyle's choice of words here indicates that he is thinking of the physical components as qualitatively (or more precisely) chemically different. This is less a "billiard ball" model of variously sized, identical particles in motion than it is a chemical "soup," in which moving particles change their essential qualities as they interact with other particles. For Boyle, this chemical change has a physical, not an occult, basis, but his definition is far less constrained by a strict mechanistic perspective than Descartes'. Boyle's conceptualization might be termed a "chemical dynamics" rather than a "positional dynamics." Such a physico-chemical framework afforded the possibility of some confirmation via experiment and to Boyle's mind was of much more immediate use to empirical investigators than the more rigorous but less verifiable model of Descartes. We see here that chemical explanation again is used in tandem with mechanical arguments. It is also notable that Boyle's perspective is totally qualitative rather than quantitative.

Another major difference between Boyle's perception of the body as machine and Descartes' is the scope of focus. Descartes had achieved his greatest insight into the body as a mechanism by idealizing it and displaying vital operations in their starkest mechanical simplicity, eliminating any discussion of the context in which that body existed. Boyle, however, insisted on considering the body as it interacted materially at every instant with its environment. Boyle held that particles from the external environment entered the body continually, via inspiration or simply by insinuating themselves through pores in the skin. Some of these particles, such as air (or more accurately, a particular part of air), were necessary for the sustaining of life. Other particles, once inside the body, had the potential of qualitatively modifying its composition and altering vital functions by virtue of their motion and interaction with other particles found within.[66] To eliminate a consideration of the entire context in which the body functioned was to provide only an artificial approximation of body function. For Boyle, the interesting aspect was not normal activity but *change.* Boyle's focus was on the body as a *reactive* mechanism.

Boyle felt that the body's reaction to change could and should be described in terms of corpuscular interactions. It was the alterations of the "textural configuration" of the body that manifested themselves as a varied assortment of physical symptoms. Viewing the body as a smaller integrated system within a larger system of nature was useful conceptually. It provided both the medical theorist and the practicing physician (1) a means to define health, in terms of the relative efficiency of the organism in its daily situation; (2) a rationale for the physician's active intervention, by explaining, for example, how specific substances could be introduced and rendered operative as remedies; and (3) a basis for classifying diseases, by showing how certain alterations correlated with certain symptoms.

The utility of the body-machine metaphor, Boyle believed, could in fact best be appreciated when, due to a variety of accidents, the body was put out of order, for only then, by observing the pattern of symptoms displayed, could one understand the close interdependence of otherwise seemingly unrelated parts. Boyle insisted that consideration of external environmental factors, important both to the sustaining of life and to the altering of stasis that could result in disease or death, provided important insights into biological function. Attention to the external environment, then, did not complicate one's understanding of the human body; it was essential to it.

The value for physicians of this conceptual view of the body was that it established some parameters for medical intervention. As Boyle explained in *Free Inquiry into the Vulgarly Received Notion of Nature,* "The physician (here supposed to be free from prejudices and mistakes) is to look upon his patient's body, as an engine, that is out of order, but yet is so constituted, that, by his concurrence with the endeavors, or rather the tendencies, of the parts of the automaton itself, it may be brought to a better state."[67] The conscientious healer, however, is free to intervene when the disease has altered the body to the point where malfunction continues despite any intrinsic quality of self-correction. The physician then acts to adjust the system, usually by promoting a beneficial alteration of texture by means of specific drugs, in order to restore the body to more efficient operation. A good physician must know the many ways a body can be altered. This required an understanding of a wide spectrum of causative factors. Boyle compared the body to a multistring musical instrument, which can be frequently out of tune due to the wide variety of alterations to which its multifarious parts are subject.[68] Only the physician well trained in natural philosophy could gain sufficient insights to aid recovery and alleviate pain and suffering.

Boyle's concept of the body as a machine owed as much to his commitment to the idea of a predetermined design in nature as to his appreciation of the elegance and simplicity of mechanical description. For Boyle, reflection on final causes was required for any comprehensive explanation of natural events. Given humanity's limited powers to understand God's methods and purpose, it was fitting for people to resort to the analogy of the machine to explain how the curious interplay of circumstances affected the body's everyday functioning. But Boyle was careful to emphasize that since human beings can use *reason* to maximize their own bodily welfare, they could avoid some of those alterations to which the body was subject due to naturally occurring external forces.[69] Drawing upon a traditional metaphor, Boyle maintained that the body should be viewed as a "manned boat."[70] Because of these directive elements—of divine presence, of the preordained design in nature, and of the piloting function of reason (which permitted one to make some, but not all, decisions to protect one's own life)—Boyle saw definite limitations to regarding body activity as strictly and blindly mechanical. However, Boyle was as insistent as Descartes that in general, the routine activities of the living body were explicable without reference to spiritual intermediaries or plastic principles in nature.

It is interesting to note also how Boyle's interest in the characteristics of air under different conditions of temperature and pressure carried over into his perception of the functioning of the system of the human body. He posited that the ability of the human body to resist alteration in the face of external factors was due to its overall corpuscular texture, which possessed an "elastical" quality that he termed the "motion of restitution." This motion of restitution permitted the body to regain its former configuration after it had been altered only briefly, just as a spring pulled and then soon released resumes its original shape. This is analogous to the model of elasticity Boyle had developed to explain the behavior of air under varying pressure conditions. The advantage of using this model when discussing the ability of the human body to "heal itself" was that it allowed one to explain constancy of form wholly in physical terms. The notion that the body as a system had an inherent elasticity was also used by Boyle in differentiating the state of health (as efficient function) from disease (as defective function) and from death (as lack of function). The condition of health is predicated upon the body's ability to recover its former state (or as much of its former state as possible) after external factors have caused textural changes.

Boyle found his notion of an elastical quality as an inherent feature of the body texture particularly useful in medical explanation. For him it replaced the Galenic model of qualitative humoral equilibrium, which had guided the traditional *methodus medendi.* Boyle tried to treat this elastical quality in a totally mechanical fashion, but as in the case of Newton's gravity, its cause was unintelligible save as an element of divine design. For Boyle this notion of elasticity became a fundamental concept in his medical thought, allowing him to explain some of the unique characteristics of living beings without espousing a vitalist position. The cause of elasticity might not be derivable from strict mechanical laws, but it did not require the postulation of a sentient force either. Elasticity was not an intrinsic property of matter but a characteristic of the dynamics of the system as a whole. Thus its operations were amenable to mechanical explanation. The complex events relating to disease could still be interpreted, then, within the basic framework of the corpuscular hypothesis.

Despite his belief in the utility of the body-machine concept, Boyle recognized some definite limitations to the *application* of the model. Sensation posed a special challenge to mechanical interpretation, for Boyle no less than for Descartes. Boyle's solution to this problem was to reject the possibility of ever describing sensation by strict mechanical laws and to devise a new category of operations, which he called "supra-mechanical," for that purpose. Supra-mechanical actions were regular and predictable insofar as they were part of a preestablished design in nature, but they differed both from supernatural operations, which are not constrained by divine design, and from mechanical explanation, since they could not fully be explicated or produced simply by the motion of material particles.[71] This is not to suggest that at some point in the future, when the mechanisms of nature were better established, a mechanical explanation of even this category of operations could be articulated. For the present, however, Boyle did not feel that the exclusion of explanations of sensory phenomena compromised the utility of the analogy of the body-machine in general.

To summarize, it appears that Boyle and Descartes promoted the notion of the body as machine for different ends. Descartes' rigorous articulation of the body-machine model brought it into sharp focus for the first time as a conceptual tool. This was his conscious intent. Descartes' might be called the classic mechanistic conception of the body, one that reveals the explanatory power of the mechanical philosophy. Boyle was less interested in articulating the idea of the body as a perfectly mechanical self-contained system than he was in illustrating how the living body reacted with the external world and how both were ultimately part of a single dynamic system, designed by God. The relevance of Boyle's model of the body as a hydraulico-pneumatic engine to medical thought was that it offered a conceptual framework for visualizing disease, testing new remedies (and verifying old ones), and generating new hypotheses—all without recourse to occult explanation. In Boyle's effort to achieve a meaningful, wholly physical explanation he tended to pass over some of the knottier questions about the nature of organic matter (such as irritability), which were to be argued far more extensively by eighteenth-century theorists in dealing with the mind-body problem. Nonetheless, the views Boyle developed on the body-machine served their purpose within his broader philosophy and afforded (or so he thought) useful clues to the physician.

Boyle's corpuscular perspective offered a way to synthesize a variety of information about both observable events and events beyond the purview of the senses, whether regarding animate or inanimate bodies in nature. By establishing levels of hypothesis, Boyle allowed for the development of intermediate theories that could extend human knowledge without requiring that lower-level hypotheses be reduced to strictly mechanical principles. Yet the assumption was that nature was orderly and did in fact operate by simple and consistent mechanical laws, even if human researchers could only partly articulate how this happened. Chemistry was an important means of both gaining immediate insights into nature and displaying the overall value of the corpuscular hypothesis.

Boyle insisted that no scientific explanations, not even the most compelling, should be treated as certain. Thus he hoped to avoid premature system building and dogmatism. This probabilism should not be seen, however, as a weakness of his approach to science. As Christoph Meinel has asserted in a recent evaluation of the empirical support for the corpuscular theory, its tentative nature made the corpuscular hypothesis more viable than "any rigid theory or ontological determination ever would have been. Its directing influence on future research was founded less on immediate results, than . . . on the basis of hope and promise."[72] It is this optimism that investigators could improve scientific understanding without first solidifying their notions of how nature really works at its most basic level that legitimizes Boyle's experimental program.

"Divulging of Useful Truths in Physick"

CHAPTER THREE

The Augmentation of Medical Knowledge

Boyle hoped that his experimental methodology, aided conceptually by the corpuscular hypothesis and his model of the body as a machine that interacted with its external environment, would lead to a better understanding of health and disease. Boyle insisted that investigations be conducted in an open, collaborative environment. He recognized that an understanding of the body in its various manifestations of health and disease required investigation from several perspectives, and he viewed anatomical study, physiological experimentation (such as that he and his colleagues had engaged in at Oxford), and chemical analysis as especially useful.

The specific biomedical topics under investigation at Oxford in the 1650s and 1660s influenced Boyle's ideas on the type of research that would be most useful for improving medicine. Much of the tone for this research had been set by William Harvey, whose discovery of the circulation of the blood necessitated a revision of many traditional medical concepts. Boyle's interest in chemistry and new drug therapies led him to focus on the chemical aspects of human physiology and of drug action, areas Harvey had not particularly emphasized.

The efforts of Boyle and other virtuosi to investigate biomedical phenomena came at a time when professional medicine was beleaguered by competition from unlicensed practitioners. In London the Royal College of Physicians, insecure about its political support in this period of civil discord and finding itself incapable of enforcing controls over medical practice, actually shifted to a more accommodating attitude regarding nontraditional medical ideas. Although this more open-minded outlook may have been prompted largely by the need to quell rampant criticism of the College and restore its credibility, it is also true that a number of members of the College, particularly some of the younger members, were interested in investigating some of the newer ideas being forwarded. The danger was in capitulating too much, for approving the elements of practice of unlicensed practitioners would undermine the stature of the medical professional.

Therefore, Boyle's unabashed call for a new, consciously eclectic modus operandi for medical investigation was not something all professional physicians were particularly anxious to embrace. Boyle insisted, nonetheless, that only by admitting a broadened knowledge base could medicine become an integral part of the overall scientific enterprise. The benefit to physicians, Boyle felt, would be the improvement of the existing *methodus medendi.*

Anatomy as a Visual Tool

As noted above, it was the challenge of investigating the implications of Harvey's discovery of blood circulation that most united the Oxford researchers.[1] These men not only attempted to emulate Harvey's methods; they saw their own work as completing the reappraisal of physiological operations that Harvey had begun. Boyle arrived at Oxford already possessed of the skills in anatomy requisite for studies of this type. He became a significant collaborator and eventually mentor in the group's work.

On the most basic level, the physiological investigations being done at Oxford required researchers to have a good knowledge of both human and comparative anatomy and skill in dissection. Although the study of gross anatomy had progressed considerably since the Renaissance, the usefulness of anatomy in extending the boundaries of medical knowledge was by no means universally accepted. Chemists, for example, did not believe that anatomical study could contribute to an understanding of physiological functions, which they saw as ultimately chemical. Those who espoused a more empirical methodology, such as the physician Thomas Sydenham, would argue that progress in medicine could be achieved only through the accumulation of clinical data directly appropriate to the physician's craft. While almost everyone agreed that a basic understanding of anatomy was useful, many held that detailed anatomical investigation, though interesting, rendered no practical benefit to the physician, since insights into function could never be attained by an investigation of structure alone. In vitro investigations were thought to be particularly limited in value, since they provided no appreciation whatsoever of the body's constitution in vivo.

Harvey's work, however, had shown that vivisection could reveal significant clues about how the body worked. Harvey's genius, in fact, was to use evidence derived from carefully devised vivisection experiments to prove his circulation theory. This method was a new tool for visualizing the body, allowing the relation of structure to function to be tangibly illustrated. The opportunity to gain insights into how the body operated while alive was sufficiently intriguing to encourage the Oxford investigators to investigate further.[2]

The notion of the body as an integrated whole consisting of organized moving parts, that is, the view of the human body as a physical *system,* became the conceptual paradigm for physiological study. For Boyle, this conceptualization might well have had much broader religious and social ramifications. Not only did it highlight the profound complexity of the body, thus putting the observer in awe of the Creator, but it served, by analogy, to indicate how society itself might flourish by active and harmonious cooperation of its members.

Boyle found it especially intriguing to join his new Oxford colleagues in more detailed investigations of the human body. He had been introduced to anatomy by two of the best anatomists in England—William Petty and Nathaniel Highmore—before coming to Oxford. Further, while living at Stalbridge, Boyle had been kept well-informed of the latest anatomical publications coming from the Continent by his friend and mentor Thomas Hartlib. Since Boyle preferred to advance science through practical demonstration, not rough speculative arguments, he was quick to appreciate that the visual clues to the workings of the human body obtained through anatomical investigation afforded a powerful means for improving the physician's understanding.

Boyle asserted that a basic knowledge of anatomy was essential not only for the practicing physician but for anyone who sought to know nature. In part 1 of the *Usefulness of Experimental Natural Philosophy,* Boyle argues that no one should shun such activity as distasteful, since "whatever God himself has been pleased to think worthy his making, its fellow-creature man should not think unworthy of his knowing."[3] The dimension of religious edification was clearly noted in the *Appendix to the Second Part of the Christian Virtuoso,* where Boyle enumerates the "anatomy of a dead body" among those things the virtuoso should investigate, because the "contemplation of [such subjects] may conduce to piety, and suggest reflections fit to excite and cherish devotion."[4] This latter work, written late in Boyle's life, shows his consistency in relating the general study of anatomy to his larger agenda of reading the Book of Nature.

But Boyle realized that the greatest practical advantage of the general study of anatomy was to the physician. In part 2 of *Usefulness of Experi-*

mental Natural Philosophy, he delineates specific instances where anatomical investigation, whether by nonmedical researchers or professional physicians, could augment medical knowledge, if not aid in medical reform.

Although Galen himself had been a skilled anatomist, in its medieval Scholastic form, Galenic medicine had come to rely more on established theory than on direct observation. Diagnosis was based on the time-honored Galenic notion of ill-health as systemic disequilibrium (manifested as an imbalance of the humors in the body). The physician was to determine the degree of systemic malfunction by external examination, such as changes in color or amount of excretions or fever and the patient's own description of his or her malaise. Reading the accepted authoritative works in medicine would provide most of the information the physician needed. Anatomy was viewed as more indispensable to the surgeon than to the physician. Although considerable anatomical work was done during the Renaissance, even by the seventeenth century many physicians still viewed anatomical dissection as less important than book learning.

For Boyle, however, anatomical observation served a fundamental pictorial purpose: it allowed the observer to see the interrelationship of solid and fluid parts. In Boyle's mature thought, the human body was described as a hydraulico-pneumatic machine subject to alterations produced by matter in motion. The study of anatomy was an important first step in viewing the body as a dynamic whole. Anatomical investigation also provided insights into how alterations affecting one part of the body could result in illness or how a specific drug aimed at a localized body part could restore health, which made it of primary importance to the physician.

Although the iatrochemists also had viewed the body as a system, for them the body comprised a *chemical* system, so knowledge of gross anatomy was relatively less important. Since Boyle's conceptual model was part chemical and part mechanistic, it was just as important to understand the structure of the solid parts of the body as it was to understand body fluids.

The importance Boyle placed on anatomical investigation as a learning tool is evident in the interest he began to take, while at Oxford, in techniques for preserving anatomical specimens. Preserving anatomical specimens for more than a few days would make them more widely available and would make more detailed investigations possible. Boyle noted that "it cannot but be a great help to the student of anatomy to be able to preserve the parts of human bodies, and those of other animals . . . so long, that he may have recourse to them at pleasure, and contemplate each of them so often and so considerately, till he have taken sufficient notice of the shape, situation, connection, etc. of the vessel, bone, or other part, and firmly impressed an idea of it upon his memory."[5] The preservation of soft tissue along with bone was preferable, Boyle maintained, since this helped the physician to visualize the placement of the organs of the body more clearly.

Preservation of specimens was not a simple matter in Boyle's time. However, using his extensive chemical knowledge, Boyle was able to develop a preservative based on turpentine that was useful in preserving small specimens. In *Usefulness of Experimental Natural Philosophy* he provides a rather long discussion on how to improve specimen preservation and emphasizes that this is a good example of how the (chemically) trained natural philosopher very tangibly could benefit the physician.[6]

Boyle was intrigued by the work of several men who claimed a particular ability to lay out preserved anatomical parts so as to show their proper spatial relationship. Such techniques would not only enhance understanding of the location of organs but provide important clues to how disease might spread within the body. Boyle personally sponsored the English translation in 1659 of "A Tract touching the skill of a better way of Anatomy of Man's Body," by the Belgian Louis de Bils. De Bils claimed to have developed a process for preserving human cadavers with all internal organs (except for the "guts and brains") still in place—the standard procedure required the immediate removal of the internal organs to prevent putrefaction. Boyle commissioned John Pell to translate the work and personally paid for the costs of printing it. The finished translation was distributed by Hartlib.[7]

If Boyle felt that the first step in understanding the organization of the human body was to know basic human anatomy, he also recognized the value of comparative anatomy to the physician. Boyle pointed out, as an example, that "the discoveries of the milky vessels in the mesentery by Asellius, of those in the thorax by Pecquet, and of the *basa lymphatica* by Bartholinus, were first made in brute bodies, though afterwards found to hold in human ones."[8] Comparative anatomy could be useful also in solving anatomical controversies:

> For as in general it is scarce possible to learn the true nature of any creature, from the consideration of the single creature it self; so particularly of divers parts of an human body it is very difficult to learn the true use, without consulting the bodies of other animals, wherein the parts inquired after

is by nature either wholly left out as needless, or wherein its differing bigness, or situation, or figure, or connection with, and relation to other parts, may render its use more conspicuous, or at least, more discernible.[9]

An understanding of animal anatomy was also necessary for the training of those who wished to engage in experimentation in vivo. After all, one needed to know what structures existed and where they were located before one could design any meaningful in vivo experiment. In vivo experimentation was the necessary second step in revealing the dynamics of the human body. Certainly it was Harvey's work that initially inspired such thinking. In part 2 of *Usefulness of Experimental Natural Philosophy,* written during his stay at Oxford, Boyle noted the great value of vivisection, explaining that "divers things in anatomy, as particularly the motion of the blood and chyle, cannot be discovered in a dead dissected body (where the cold hath shut up and obliterated many passages) that may be seen in one opened alive."[10] Boyle felt that the significant information obtainable through vivisection justified the use of animal experimentation for this purpose.[11]

Researchers at Oxford in the mid-seventeenth century came to utilize in vivo experimental techniques extensively in their efforts to discern the purpose of respiration and to investigate how the circulating blood might carry drug substances through the body. Boyle became actively involved in this type of inquiry. His work using the air pump to conduct in vivo experiments on respiration contributed significantly to the overall research effort. By enclosing the living animal in an evacuated receiver (thus confining it to an environmental "system" with definable and measurable variables), one could obtain insights into how the "system" of the living body was affected by the larger system of its environment.

Physiological Experimentation

In vivo experiments could also shed light on specific physiological functions. Boyle's work on respiration is one example of this. His active participation in the work on respiration done at Oxford in the 1650s and 1660s also provided an opportunity for him to see firsthand the benefits of collaboration on a scientific problem. A review of the work of Boyle and his colleagues on respiration also reveals how closely intertwined was Boyle's medical work with his other scientific interests.

Boyle's contributions to the research into respiration at Oxford are distinguished not only by the careful way he planned experiments but by his willingness to utilize new tools to extend the scope of investigation. Many new scientific instruments had come into use during the Scientific Revolution. As I noted above, Boyle readily welcomed devices such as the microscope. The air pump, developed by Boyle's capable colleague and lab assistant, Robert Hooke, was to prove especially valuable in experiments to determine the role of the air in maintaining life and the possible relationship between the processes of respiration and combustion.

The initial stimulus to the inquiry into respiration at Oxford had come also from William Harvey. Harvey's work on blood circulation had cast doubt on the traditional Galenic explanation that air was brought from the lungs by the pulmonary veins to the left ventricle of the heart and there mixed with blood to produce vital spirit. Harvey held that vital spirit was intrinsic to the blood and that air played no role in its production. For Harvey, the purpose of respiration was to cool the blood as it passed through the lungs.[12] For this to occur, no air had to be transported by the pulmonary veins.

As Frank relates in his survey of the physiological work at Oxford in the seventeenth century, two problems remained to be solved by Harvey's successors. First, if air does not enter the body, why is it needed? And second, how can one explain the change of venous blood into arterial if one dismisses the notion of a "vivifying" process involving the generation of vital spirits?[13] Numerous in vivo experiments were conducted to discover the answers. The subject was also considered from a chemical perspective. Boyle became closely involved in this work, not only sharing his own insights, replicating some of his colleagues' experiments, and helping to evaluate the various theories posited but also designing and conducting a number of in vivo experiments using the air pump to test effects on the organism of having air partially or totally evacuated.

Boyle took up the question of respiration quite early and in considerable detail. In his very first signed scientific publication, *New Experiments, Physico-Mechanical, touching the Spring of the Air* (1660), he included a long digression on the subject in the section following experiment 41.[14] He informed his readers that he had as yet performed too few experiments to draw any firm conclusions regarding the function of respiration but that he would, nonetheless, set forth his suggestions concerning how his newly contrived air pump might advance understanding of the subject.

Boyle first addressed the anatomical aspects of respiration, beginning with the arguments on whether the lungs move themselves or are moved by the thorax or the diaphragm. From his own experiments and those of Highmore, which showed that lung action ceases when the thorax stops moving, Boyle concluded that the diaphragm seems to be the "principal instrument of ordinary and gentle respiration." To the question what conveys air into the lungs, Boyle provided an answer based on the idea of inequality of air pressure: "Upon the bare dilation of the thorax, the spring of that internal air, or halituous substance that is wont to possess as much of the cavity of the chest as the lungs fill not up, being much weakened, the external and contiguous air must necessarily press in at the open wind-pipe into the lungs, as finding there less resistance than any where else about it."

Boyle then turned to the physiological interpretations of respiration, basing his comments on what he had observed happening to small animals in his vacuum receiver. To the argument that the function of respiration is to cool the heat of the heart, he provided several objections: (1) even cold-blooded creatures have need of respiration; (2) the best breathing air is not cold air, which one would expect to cool the vital heat more efficiently, but temperate air; and (3) the heat of the heart is a gentle heat, not a burning heat, and therefore does not appear to require constant cooling. Experimentally he had observed, in addition, that "it appears not that in our exhausted receiver, where yet animals die so suddenly for want of respiration, the ambient body is sensibly hotter than the common air." As to the argument that the purpose of respiration is to generate spirits in the heart, the view common to Galenic thought but opposed by Harvey, Boyle used the evidence of dissections to assert that air does not seem to be conveyed into the heart, and he further noted that air particles and spirits have few similar characteristics.

He next took up the argument, also forwarded by Galen, that a purpose of respiration is the removal of sooty wastes. He noted two ways in which this removal process might occur: either (1) air in the blood provides "an ambient body of a yielding nature, to receive into it the superfluous serosities, and other recrements of the blood," or (2) air reaching the end of the *aspera arteria* close to the surface of the circulating blood unites with and carries off excreta with itself when exhaled.

Concerning the first interpretation, which essentially involves the idea that air provides a space for pent-up wastes to go, Boyle argued that when air was removed from his vacuum receiver, even more space was created for the excreta to be received, but since the animal died, this explanation of what happens in respiration was invalid. Concerning the second interpretation, that excreted waste particles unite with air particles and are exhaled together, Boyle said that this was consistent with the suggestion that "there is a certain consistence of air requisite to respiration: so that if it be too thick, and already overcharged with vapours, it will be unfit to unite with, and carry off those of the blood . . . and if it be too thin. . . , the number or size of the aerial particles is too small to be able to carry off the halituous excrements of the blood in such plenty as is requisite." That air can become too thick for respiration is shown by the experiences of miners stifled by the thick air in mines, and by Boyle's own experiment upon a bird who was suffocated in a small receiver by its own exhalations. That rarefied air also is unfit for adequate respiration is shown by the experiences of men climbing to high altitudes. Boyle, therefore, would allow the argument that sooty wastes were removed by respiration, provided the process of that removal was explained according to the second of his two cited interpretations.

Boyle suspected, however, that air does more than just remove superfluities from the blood. He quoted Paracelsus's statement "that as the stomach concocts meat, and makes part of it useful to the body, rejecting the other part; so the lungs consume part of the air, and proscribe the rest." Boyle, like some of his Oxford contemporaries, was willing to conjecture that only a part of the air might be utilized in respiration. At this stage in the development of his thought, Boyle did not try to define this part of the air, except to characterize it, in a manner consistent with his early iatrochemical training, as a "vital quintessence . . . which, [since it] serves to the refreshment and restauration of our vital spirits for which use the grosser and incomparably greater part of the air being unserviceable, it need not seem strange, that an animal stands in need of almost incessantly drawing in fresh air." Boyle, with customary caution, refused to speculate on the exact chemical nature of this "quintessence"; however, it is clear that he considered it material.

Boyle admitted that very little was understood about how air physically was utilized, noting his earlier objections to the idea that air generates vital spirits and his inability to perceive how air was translated into increased heat. Yet at this point his own observations of both the expiration of life and of flame in his vacuum receiver caused him to maintain that "our engine thus shews us a new kind of resemblance betwixt fire and life" and to agree with those who believed that air was necessary to "cherish the vital flame, which they do suppose to be continually burning in the heart." Boyle ended this section by providing several observations illustrating that all animals need air.[15]

Boyle concluded with the following summary:

> Without denying then, that the inspired and exspired air may be sometimes very useful, by condensing and cooling the blood that passeth through the lungs; I hold that the depuration of the blood in that passage, is not only one of the ordinary, but one of the principal uses of respiration.

> But I am apt also to suspect, that the air doth something else in respiration, which hath not yet been sufficiently explained.[16]

Boyle also brought his knowledge of chemistry to bear on his inquiries into respiration. Like some of his Oxford colleagues, he took up the question whether a "nitrous substance" in air was that specific component necessary to life. The physiologists working at Oxford in the 1650s and 1660s were intrigued by the possibility that a single nitrous substance in the air "fed" both life and flame.[17] Niter (potassium nitrate) was a substance well known to chemists, since it was a powerful oxidizing agent. Boyle himself had performed experiments on it while associated with Benjamin Worsley in the early days of the Invisible College. He recognized its heating and cooling properties and its practical use (as a fertilizer and as an essential ingredient in gunpowder). The potency of this substance made it a prime subject for alchemical speculation. The idea of an *aerial* niter that played a role in sustaining life and combustion was first forwarded by Paracelsus and elaborated upon by the alchemists Alexander Seton and Michael Sendivogius (of whom Boyle thought highly).[18] Kenelm Digby, also had speculated on it.[19] In the early 1660s Boyle's laboratory assistant and close colleague Robert Hooke began his own investigation of the "aerial niter." Hooke saw niter and air as containing a common substance that dissolved the sulfur of a burning body. He elaborated this concept of niter as a solvent in his *Micrographia,* of 1665. Hooke extended this interpretation of niter to the process of respiration in 1667, when he informed the Royal Society that he believed there existed a nitrous quality in the air that was responsible for sustaining life. Once this nitrous component of the air became either "spent" or "clogged" by combining with gross vapors, it was rendered unfit.[20]

In 1669 Richard Lower, another Oxford researcher with whom Boyle had previously collaborated, published his findings that venous blood changes color in its passage through the lungs. Lower speculated that the "nitrous spirit" in the air was the cause of this color change.[21] He did not, however, connect this uptake of nitrous spirit with the maintenance of vital heat, as Thomas Willis was soon to do.

Willis, whose work displays an interesting blend of iatrochemical and corpuscular ideas, had also long investigated the subject of niter and combustion. In 1670, influenced by the work of both Hooke and Lower, he published his own views on respiration. Willis saw life itself as a kind of flame, and he suggested that the purpose of respiration was to kindle that flame by bringing the niter of the air into the body, where it volatilized the sulfur of the blood.[22]

"Divulging of Useful Truths in Physick"

Boyle had briefly considered whether the air played a role in the crystallization or artificial production of niter in a section of his *Certain Physiological Essays,* of 1661, entitled "A Physico-Chymical Essay containing an Experiment relating to Salt-Petre." This experiment, in general, involved the separation and recomposition of niter. It reveals that Boyle was well aware of the fixed and volatile components of this substance. However, with regard to the air, although he suggested that air "so enriched with variety of steams from terrestrial (not here to determine whether it receive not some also from celestial) bodies" could produce chemical change, he admitted that he could not then draw concrete conclusions specifically regarding the presence of niter in the air itself.[23]

In the early 1670s, Boyle performed a series of additional respiration experiments. In his "New Pneumatical Experiments about Respiration: A Continuation," title 15, published in *Philosophical Transactions,* 12 September 1670, Boyle attempted to determine whether a loss of air could be detected after its respirable component was used up. He placed a mouse in a closed receiver, along with a mercury gauge to measure air pressure. After the mouse had suffocated (i.e., when it supposedly had utilized all the respirable part of the air in the receiver), he compared the air pressure reading against the original reading; there was no change.[24] This lack of evidence that air was used up in respiration hurt Hooke's theory, for he had suggested that air and niter contained a common component, the loss of which should be detectable in both combustion and respiration. Boyle, for whom the most manifest characteristic of air was the "spring" of its particles, found that his mercury gauge measured no loss of "spring."[25] The substance utilized in respiration, therefore, was not, as Hooke had postulated, a component of air. (This did not, however, preclude the possibility that something carried *along with* the air was being utilized in combustion and respiration.)

In his *New Experiments touching the Relation betwixt Flame and Air,* of 1672, Boyle specifically considered the necessity of air to combustion. He performed several experiments in his vacuum receiver to illustrate that in the absence of air, inflammable substances would not ignite. He found that even gunpowder, despite its "great disposition to take fire," would not ignite in the receiver.[26] A further experiment revealed, however, that once ignited, gunpowder would keep burning under water. Boyle cautioned those who would take this result as proof that air was unnecessary in some combustions by positing that (1) air might indeed have been present in the pores of the water (a suggestion he believed to be true on the basis of some earlier experiments)[27] or (2) the corpuscles of saltpeter themselves had "intercepted" a store of aerial particles, which allowed for the continued combustion.[28] These experiments brought doubt upon Hooke's contention that niter could independently support combustion. They also show that Boyle at this point preferred to visualize air as "physically enclosed" in saltpeter rather than chemically combined with it.[29]

In his *New Experiments about the Relation betwixt Air and the Flamma Vitalis of Animals,* published in 1672, Boyle considered the necessity of air to life and attempted to determine by experiment the existence of the vital flame. Boyle measured the weight of a mouse in a receiver before and after death to see whether a weight increase could be detected after the expiration of the vital flame (which according to the Aristotelian interpretation should possess levity). It could not. He also placed glowworms (whose luminosity was thought to be a visible manifestation of the vital flame) in a receiver to see whether they ceased to glow when the air was removed and found that they did. In a nice example of a controlled experiment, he placed silkworm eggs in two receivers and exhausted the air from one to determine whether they needed air to hatch; he found evidence to indicate that the "seminal rudiments" needed air in order to be actuated.[30]

The most important experiments reported in this particular treatise, however, were those designed to compare the necessity of air to life with the necessity of air to combustion. He found that animals could survive longer than a kindled flame when placed in the same closed receiver. Since animals were breathing air already useless to flame, Boyle had to consider the possibility that there were actually two separate substances in the air, one supporting life and another supporting combustion. He suggested the following possibilities: (1) two separate substances were necessary for respiration and combustion; (2) a single substance was indeed utilized in both, except that common flame utilized it more wastefully and thus expired first, while the animal, requiring the maintenance of a more temperate heat, could still utilize what was left; (3) the correct interpretation was a combination of these two former suggestions; (4) some hitherto unconsidered factor played a role. Boyle was unable to ascertain the best hypothesis on the basis of available evidence, illustrating again the truth of a comment he had made many years earlier, that his researches "have made respiration appear to me rather a more, than a less mysterious thing, than it did before."[31] He was thus unwilling to follow those of his Oxford colleagues who were at this time coming more and more to maintain the existence of an aerial niter that was used up in both respiration and combustion. However compelling this idea might be from a chemical perspective, the inability of his pneumatical experiments to verify this made Boyle cautious. Here is an excellent example of Boyle's analyzing a problem from several different perspectives before rendering any conclusion.

Boyle's frustration at being unable to isolate the factor that made air so necessary for life and flame is best revealed in his 1674 work *Suspicions about some Hidden Qualities of the Air.* He believed that air was a composite substance with a variety of corpuscular constituents whose identities had not yet been ascertained; nor could it *ever* be capable of a full analysis, given that the actual composition varied in accordance with time and place. In his words, air was "not, as many imagine, a simple and elementary body, but a confused aggregate of effluviums from such differing bodies, that, tho they all agree in constituting, by their minuteness and various motions, one great mass of fluid matter, yet perhaps there is scarce a more heterogeneous body in the world."[32] Boyle had determined that the "most genuine and distinguishing property" of the air, its "spring," was not lost after the air became unfit for combustion and respiration. Nor could Boyle detect any other visible alteration of the air after its invigorating component was used up. "And indeed," he remarked, "it seems to deserve our wonder, what that should be in the air, which enabling it to keep flame, does yet, by being consumed or depraved, so suddenly render the air unfit to make flame subsist. And it seems by the sudden wasting or spoiling of this fine subject, whatever it be, that the bulk of it is but very small in proportion to the air it impregnates with its virtue."[33]

Since Boyle refused to speculate on specifically what this ingredient of air was, he was forced, despite his aversion to occult concepts, to explain his findings in the following vague terms:

> The difficulty we find of keeping flame and fire alive, tho but for a little time, without air, makes me sometimes prone to suspect, that there may be dispersed through the rest of the atmosphere some odd substance, either of a solar, or astral, or some other exotic nature, on whose account the air is so necessary to the subsistence of flame; which necessity I have found to be greater, and less dependent upon the manifest attributes of the air, than naturalists seem to have observed.[34]

He further shows an unwillingness to drop the subject of the similarities between respiration and combustion, even though he could find no evidence to support the theory of an aerial niter being consumed in both processes. But because of the limited state of knowledge about the subject, his cautious nature would allow him was to suggest only "a great suspicion of some vital substance, if I may so call it, diffused through the air, whether it be a volatile niter, or (rather) some yet anonimous substance, sydereal or subterraneal, but not improbably of kin to that, which I lately noted to be so necessary to the maintenance of other flames."[35]

In 1674 John Mayow, who himself was much indebted to Boyle's pioneer work on respiration, published his *Tractatus Quinque,* in which he forwarded new evidence that air in fact was altered in the process of respiration. He first suggested that the air owes its spring to the springy particles of a nitroaerial spirit, which are linked to air particles. He then revealed that he had experimentally detected a loss of spring when respirable air was used up. Mayow was able to achieve this by designing his experiment differently from Boyle's.

Mayow placed a burning candle into a cupping glass and inverted it in a container of water. The water levels were equalized inside and outside the cupping glass. When the candle burned out, it was observed that the inside water level had risen, giving credence to the hypothesis that the air in the glass had lost some elasticity. Boyle's method had utilized a closed receiver, which had concealed the decrease Mayow had observed.[36] Ironically, it was Boyle's procedure that was more accurate: the observed "loss of air elasticity" in Mayow's experiment was really due to the fact that the gaseous products of combustion (which no one at that time could have correctly identified) had dissolved in the water.

Using his "evidence," Mayow concluded that sulfur particles escaped from a burning or respiring body to dislodge the nitroaerial particles in the air, with the result that the air lost its spring. Combining his knowledge of chemistry with mechanical notions, Mayow equated this reciprocal agitation of the nitroaerial and saline-sulphureous particles with fermentation, which generated heat. Mayow saw the processes of respiration and combustion as involving, not consumption of a given component of the air, but the destruction of a force of elasticity. The "force" or spirit that made air elastic was that force or spirit that sustained life or flame. Richard Westfall interprets this model as treating nitroaerial particles as if they were Hermetic active principles.[37]

Boyle was not satisfied with Mayow's interpretation. First, Boyle was convinced that his own experimental design was sound and that if there was a loss of spring, then he too should have observed it. Second, Boyle's extensive past experiments on saltpeter had revealed to him that that substance possessed chemical qualities inconsistent with the supposed nature of a nitroaerial component of the air. His specific arguments against the nitroaerial hypothesis are set forth in his posthumously published *History of the Air* (1691), under title 11:

> I know, that divers learned men . . . speak much of a volatile niter, that abounds in the air, as if that were the only salt wherewith it is impreg-

nated. But though I agree with them, in thinking, that the air is in many places impregnated with corpuscles of a nitrous nature; yet I confess I have not been hitherto convinced of all that is wont to be delivered about the plenty and quality of the niter in the air: for I have not found, that those, that build so much upon this volatile niter, have made out by any competent experiment, that there is such a volatile niter abounding in the air. For having often dealt with salt-petre in the fire, I do not find it easy to be raised by a gentle heat; and when by a stronger fire we distil it in close vessels, it is plain, that what the chemists call spirit of niter, has quite differing properties from crude niter, and from those that are ascribed to the volatile niter of the air; these spirits being so far from being refreshing to the nature of animals, that they are exceeding corrosive.[38]

Boyle nonetheless remained characteristically open-minded about the subject, adding that perhaps the action of sunbeams and various subterraneal exhalations on niter in the air volatilizes it differently from the fires in his laboratory. If this were so, naturally volatilized niter would have different chemical characteristics than the niter he had worked with in the lab. But still he pointed out that even if air did contain niter, it contained many other salts as well, which indicated that investigators would be hard put to show that it was specifically a nitrous salt that was present commonly and in sufficient supply to perform the functions attributed to it.[39]

Boyle had no alternative hypothesis to offer. Therefore, he closed his discussion of the matter by calling the aerial niter hypothesis "an ingenious supposition" that might at some future time be shown to have some validity.[40] Since scientific inquiry was to be an ongoing activity, Boyle saw nothing wrong with leaving this particular hypothesis, as so many others dealing with something as complex as life had been left, unresolved.

Boyle's work in pneumatics caused him to turn his attention to a physical conceptualization of air. He became interested, among other things, in the role of the air as a medium of transport for effluvial particles that sloughed off from earthly substances and were dispersed widely thereby. Boyle suggested that the air might act as a menstruum to change the constitution of some of these particles. He suggested that attention be given to how these particles (in altered or unaltered form) might enter the human body to produce changes. This line of thinking, which had special ramifications for medical thought, is investigated more fully in chapter 4.

Although Boyle's own research into the subject of respiration led him to reject his colleagues' chemical conclusions concerning the aerial niter, he never veered from his belief that chemical investigation was a major way to obtain information and generate hypotheses valuable to medicine. In fact, it was his own considerable chemical facility, which permitted him to obtain extensive knowledge of the properties of niter, that caused him to reject the particular chemical hypothesis (of niter as the active substance involved in respiration) espoused by his associates.

Boyle continued his chemical investigations both while at Oxford and afterwards in London. Part 2 of *Usefulness of Experimental Natural Philosophy*, in which his beliefs on how the physician might profit from a broader scientific perspective are outlined, is full of comments on just how profitable chemical knowledge could be. Boyle felt specifically that chemical analysis would increase one's understanding of the body humors, on which so much of traditional therapeutics had been based. Referring to the debates, quite vocal in his day, criticizing Galenic ideas, Boyle remarked with his customary caution that although he was "very unwilling to meddle with medical controversies," he was yet "apt to think, that chymists are wont to speak somewhat too slightingly of the humours of the human body, and allow them too little a share in the production of diseases."[41]

Boyle did not reject the notions of disease promoted by the chemists in favor of traditional humoral views; he believed, however, that understanding of disease and cure could be augmented by fuller investigation into the actual composition of the humors. For Boyle, Galen's humoral perspective was deficient, based as it was on simple visual observation and the positing of occult qualities to explain changes and effects. Only by chemical analysis could a more rigorous understanding of the nature of the humors be achieved. He explained:

> And indeed, if the juices of the body were more chymically examined, especially by a naturalist, that knows the ways of making fixed bodies volatile, and volatile fixed, and knows the power of the open air in promoting the former of those operations; it is not improbable, that both many things relating to the nature of the humours, and to the ways of sweetening, actuating, and otherwise altering them, may be detected, and the importance of such discoveries may be discerned.

Chemistry could be of use in pathology, not only by providing knowledge of humoral composition but also by helping to explain disturbances such as fevers. Boyle maintained that "he, that thoroughly understands the nature of ferments and fermentations, shall probably be much better able than he, that ignores them, to give a fair account of divers phaenomena of several diseases (as well fevers as others) which will perhaps be never thoroughly understood, without an insight into the doctrine of fermentation." Yet it is clear that Boyle did not assume that all commotions in the body were strictly due to fermentation, for he went on to note that "there may be effervescences, (and perhaps periodical ones) in the blood and other juices of the body without fermentation properly so called. . . . For there may be divers other ways of begetting a preternatural heat in the blood." In this case also, the trained chemist who knows what mixtures of substances can produce heat, can be of assistance to medicine. Chemical analysis, furthermore, can be applied to "noxious juices in distempered bodies" to enhance our understanding of concretions, such as kidney stones. Chemical investigation, then, could be employed in a number of areas to help the physician explain pathological processes.

Another area where chemical knowledge could benefit medicine was prognostics. Traditional diagnosis was based on the patient's own description of symptoms and the physician's visual inspection of excreted fluids, particularly urine. Chemical analysis of these fluids would afford additional insights:

> I dare not deny but by precipitations, and some other ways, not yet vulgarly practised, of examining the urine, made by the same patient at several times, before, in, and after some notable alteration in his body, divers things (especially in fevers, and other acute diseases) relating to the state of it, may be discovered, especially if thereto be added a skilful and seasonable chymical examen of the other excrements, and vitiated substances of the patient's body.

Even the area of hygiene could be aided by chemistry, since improved cooking techniques and food preservation methods would ultimately affect the general state of health of the population. And a fuller understanding of the chemical composition and effects of various liquors that were often used as tonics could extend their medicinal uses.

The area of medicine for which chemical investigation held the most promise, however, was therapeutics. Boyle delineated several general ways in which chemical knowledge could enhance therapeutics. These include an increased appreciation of how particular substances react in the human body and the artificial creation of wholly new drugs in the laboratory (which Boyle hoped would result in new cures for currently unmanageable diseases or alternative therapies for diseases currently treated by drastic measures such as cautery and surgery). Chemical investigation could also result in improved drug quality and improved methods of drug preservation. Laboratory experimentation could lead to the development of cheaper remedies, the exposure of inefficacious ingredients, and even the modification of noxious substances so that they could be used medicinally. The result would be an improved public welfare, which Boyle held to be a key aim of his scientific program. Boyle specifically suggested that the best hope for reform of the established *methodus medendi* was the increased application of chemical knowledge to the area of therapeutics.

As noted above, Boyle used his chemical knowledge to judge the hypothesis of the role of aerial niter in respiration. His interest in chemical analysis, however, also brought him to a consideration of the chemical basis of digestion. In *Certain Physiological Essays* he related having prepared in the laboratory a substance he considered to be an imitation of digestive juice, "whereby I have in a short time, and without fire, dissociated the parts of roasted or boiled flesh, bread, fruit, etc. and . . . reduced [them] to the consistence of a fluid body."[42] Boyle believed that digestion was more than coction. He maintained that heat alone could not break down all the substances known to be digestible and asserted that the stomach was "endowed with a subtile dissolvent (whence soever it hath it) by which it may perform divers things, not to be done by . . . languid . . . heat."[43] Further evidence that the temperate body heat was insufficient to explain digestion was the existence of morbific body concretions (which Boyle interpreted in the Paracelsian manner as formed from aliments in the digestive process):

> It seems a mistake to imagine (how many soever do so) that heat must needs be efficient of all the changes the matter of our aliments may happen to undergo in a human body; where there are strainers, and solvents, and new mixtions, and perhaps ferments, and divers other powerful agents, which by successively working upon the assumed matter, may so fashion and qualify it, as in some cases, to bring the more disposed part of it to be not unlike even fossile salts, or other mineral substances.[44]

Boyle was unable to determine experimentally the specific presence of an acid in the stomach, but he held out the hope that chemistry "may not a little contribute" to an understanding of digestion. He hoped that further experiments of his own, already planned, would allow him to make conclusions concerning the existence and identity of gastric acid.[45] However, he was never able to accomplish this.[46]

Another way Boyle brought a chemical approach to the study of the human body was in his innovative work on the blood. There was great interest among physiological investigators at Oxford in the 1650s and 1660s in devising a number of experiments on blood transfusion and the injection of chemicals into the blood to see what effects could be produced on the experimental animal. Boyle added his expertise to this effort. In 1658 he informed Hartlib of "a new anatomy experimented at Oxford to open veins and sprout medicines into it."[47] He witnessed his friend Christopher Wren's first transfusion experiments at about this time.[48] In 1666 Boyle communicated to the Royal Society information on the transfusion of blood from one live dog to another, an experiment devised by Richard Lower. Boyle included comments about similar trials he had made on transfusing blood into dogs, although he had not yet transfused directly from one dog to another, and suggested how Lower's technique might be improved.[49] Shortly after this, Boyle published additional proposals and queries regarding the transfusion experiments on dogs. He suggested that various evaluations and analyses be made in transfusion experiments to detect such things as behavioral changes, changes in excreta, effects of medication (injected along with the blood), and transference of disease.[50]

While at Oxford, Boyle had engaged in chemical experiments to investigate color changes that occurred in the blood when volatile or acid salts were added. This interest in color changes in the blood was prompted by the speculations concerning aerial niter. Frank suggests that these preliminary chemical experiments led Boyle to develop a schema for research specifically on the blood and that he most likely circulated his schema at Oxford for the benefit of those who might wish to undertake such investigations.[51] Much later, in 1683, at the urging of John Locke, Boyle published his notes as *Memoirs for the Natural History of Humane Blood.* Included therein is a prospectus for a comprehensive treatment of the subject, along with some preliminary experimental observations. Boyle proposes, among other things, that a determination be made of the proportion of various substances chemically obtainable from the blood, the specific gravity of the blood, the effects of various chemicals upon the blood, the chemical characteristics of both the fibrous and serous parts of the blood (considered separately), and the medicinal uses of spirit of blood (i.e., ammonia), which Boyle held to be "one of the noblest of urinous or volatile alcalies."

By the time *Natural History of Human Blood* was published, Boyle was too ill to engage in any new extensive experiments on the subject. However, this treatise immediately caught the attention of Marcello Malpighi, who in 1686 requested Carlo Antonio Ronchi, his English contact, to discuss with Boyle the composition of the blood, as he wished to learn from Boyle whether "all [the discernible] parts are necessary for the normal composition of the blood and in what proportions, whether among them there is a successive transformation, and what he thinks is the nature of these red atometti which are found in large numbers in healthy subjects and are not evident in cachectics."[52] Malpighi evidently was interested also in obtaining specific instructions on the preparation of spirit of blood. What information Malpighi ever obtained from Boyle is unknown; Howard Adelmann cites evidence of a later letter that refers to some materials being sent but lost in transit. (The specific content of these materials is not mentioned.)

In *Natural History of Human Blood* Boyle had commented upon the idea, furthered by such men as Willis, that "inordinate fermentations in the blood" were the cause of fevers. Boyle questioned, on the basis of chemical evidence, whether true "fermentation" was actually occurring, since he could detect no presence of a "vinous or ardent spirit, though that be the usual product of fermentation in liquors." An experiment made upon blood serum alone did produce what Boyle believed to be a fermentation, yet here too the "liquor, that first ascended . . . did not taste or smell like a vinous spirit, tho it was differing from meer phlegm."[53] Given the inconclusiveness of his experimental findings, Boyle later exercised caution in referring to the movement of the blood strictly as a "fermentation," noting that he used the term in the informal sense of a "commotion" rather than as a referent to the formal chemical process.[54]

If Boyle believed that investigative techniques involving physiological experimentation and chemical analysis could vastly improve the medical art, he was even more convinced that a consideration of the larger context in which the human body operated would prove profitable to the physician. The external environment and its material impact on the "texture" of the body was of great concern to Boyle, who saw in such considerations an opportunity to utilize the conceptual power of his corpuscular hypothesis in a way that could have particular practical benefit for the improvement of the medical art.

CHAPTER FOUR

The Human Body and the Environment

It was in Boyle's articulation of how the environment affects the human body that many of his basic concepts came together as he tried to define just what was involved in the maintenance of health, the causation of disease, and the process of cure. By fusing corpuscular ideas with the assumption of a divine design in nature, Boyle was able to create a plausible holistic model of corpuscular activity that could explain function and malfunction in physical terms.

Environmental Medicine

There was considerable interest in the physical environment in Boyle's day. Clarence J. Glacken has pointed out that one of the effects of the age of discovery had been the illustration to Europeans of the many ways in which humans of different cultures shaped their environment to suit their particular needs. This realization gave new impetus to ideas in Western culture about the potential of nature to be controlled and, in Glacken's words, led to the perception "of man as a geologic or geographic agent."[1] Three main themes of the day—the idea that human beings stood at the top of the hierarchy of creation, the growing optimism over society's technological potential, and the affirmation of the work ethic which was a legacy of the Reformation—combined to produce an especially strong belief in human creative capacity to devise and implement measures to control the environment. On the more speculative level, curiosity about other peoples at this time prompted the development of theories about the role of climate and environmental influences in determining physiological temperament and thus shaping national character.[2] Considerations such as these influenced medical thought in the late seventeenth and eighteenth centuries by turning attention to how the environment could be modified to create more healthful living conditions. This led to attempts to isolate the specific environmental factors that could affect the human body.

The work of Paracelsus and Van Helmont was particularly influential in emphasizing the role of environment in health. Many medical reformers promoting iatrochemical theory came to see the investigation of environmental factors as a central feature distinguishing them from the traditionalists. Relating environmental conditions to disease was hardly a new idea in medicine, however. It not only formed a major component of Hippocratic thought but was an intrinsic part of Galenic philosophy as well. Galen had sought to extend Hippocratic ideas, and even though he focused more on the functions taking place *within* the body, his criterion for determining whether or not a body was healthy or sick was how well it functioned in relation to nature at large.[3] Nonetheless, as James C. Riley has pointed out in his investigation of the history of Enlightenment medicine, even though the idea of relating health to the environment was not new, what *was* unique in the mid-seventeenth century was that the revival of such ideas coincided with "fresh approaches to the study of man and the environment" and with a "rapidly expanding body of information about these things."[4]

Riley suggests that environmental medicine developed in three phases.[5] The first phase occurred in England from the 1660s to the 1680s. At that time, a number of virtuosi—some physicians, some not—began to correlate climatic conditions with the rise and decline of epidemics and to make detailed clinical observations that led to improved classification of diseases. Such men included Boyle, Hooke, William Petty, John Locke, Christopher Wren, and Thomas Sydenham. During the second phase, which began between 1690 and 1710, Continental writers expanded upon this work, typically engaging in more detailed, specialized investigations. By the end of the eighteenth century, researchers were faced with a growing frustration over the inability of the meteorological data so far obtained to allow accurate forecasts about coming diseases. Interest then shifted away from the idea of treating the patient to one of modifying or purging the environment of pestilential conditions. Assessing this history of environmental medicine, Riley concludes:

> In . . . the role of the environment as a source of disease, in recording the signs and symptoms of the association, in rethinking the foundations for explaining disease, and in proposing to find an efficacious medicine, the physician's thought ran parallel to the thought of students of astronomy, botany, chemistry, political institutions, criminal law, economics, and many other fields. In this realm medicine both drew from and contrib-

uted to the development of ideas, which is usually identified with the Enlightenment.[6]

Boyle's Views on Environment and Health

Although Riley discusses Boyle's contribution to this environmental trend in medical thought, most historians have not appreciated how pivotal environmental considerations are to Boyle's overall views on medicine. His investigations on the effects of the air on the human body, his support for collection of data on weather and climate, his analysis of mineral waters, and his interest in qualitative effluvia are in and of themselves revealing of an extensive fascination with the relation of the environment and health. But Boyle went even further: he used his corpuscular philosophy to provide a general explanation of how environmental factors could cause alterations in the body in wholly physical terms. Hippocrates had not provided any detailed theory of how environmental forces could affect disease and health. Paracelsus and Van Helmont had presented a theory derived from alchemical notions, yet it was one unacceptable to Boyle because of its reliance on spiritual, directive forces in nature. Boyle's views were fully integrated with the rest of his science. The study of the human body in its environmental context was to be undertaken using the same methodology as that used to investigate inanimate bodies in nature. His postulations, like the corpuscular hypothesis itself, were dependent on analogy and were couched in probabilistic terms; yet his formulations were logically consistent and forwarded with an eye to their predictive value.

Boyle's basic view was that the interaction of corpuscles was responsible for producing the various textures by which *all* material bodies were defined. Bodies in nature, however, were not isolated nor static systems; thus, they could be affected by external conditions, which could also be described in terms of corpuscular interaction. God had designed the universe as an interrelated whole. A full study of any given body in nature, then, required investigating not only the body itself as an organized system but also the external physical influences that could impinge upon it. As Boyle explained,

> We must consider each body, not barely, as it is in itself, an entire and distinct portion of matter, but as it is a part of the universe, and consequently placed among a great number and variety of other bodies, upon which it may act, and by which it may be acted on, in many ways (or upon many accounts) each of which men are wont to fancy as a distinct power or quality in the body by which those actions, or in which those passions, are pro-

duced. For if we thus consider things, we shall not much wonder that a portion of matter that is indeed endowed but with a very few mechanical affections, as such a determinate texture and motion, but is placed among a multitude of other bodies that differ in those attributes from it and one another, should be capable of having a great number and variety of relations to those other bodies, and consequently should be thought to have many distinct inherent qualities by such as look upon those several relations or respects it may have to bodies without it, as real and distinct entities implanted in the body itself.[7]

Boyle maintained that some of the qualities we perceive as intrinsic to a body are actually expressions of interactions between the body and its external environment. This was as true for simple, inanimate bodies as for more complex, organic bodies, including the human body itself.

As described in chapter 3, Boyle insisted that it was possible (and preferable) to speak of all interactions between a body and its physical environment in purely physical terms without assuming the presence of any directive force within nature itself. He insisted that "nature" was simply a "notional thing," a term of convenience used to describe "the aggregate of bodies that make up the world framed as it is." In nature so defined, all the bodies that compose it "are enabled to act upon, and fitted to suffer from one another, according to the settled laws of motion."[8]

To elucidate his ideas on how the human body specifically could be affected by external conditions of its environment, Boyle resorted to the concept, long established in Western medicine, that the human body was a "microcosm" of the larger world (the "macrocosm"). The Paracelsians had forwarded the idea that there were distinct correspondences between the macrocosm and the microcosm. Astral influences supposedly could directly affect specific parts of the body that had a spiritual identification (or correspondence) with them.

However, Boyle viewed the macrocosm and the microcosm not as linked by spiritual, directive forces but as two identifiable structural systems composed of the same material building blocks and subject to the same basic natural laws. In fact, he describes the entire "frame of the world" as encompassing such systems within systems, using the delightful metaphor of the world as a "pregnant automaton":

I consider the frame of the world already made, as a great, and if I may so speak, pregnant automaton, that, like a woman with twins in her womb, or a ship furnished with pumps, ordnance, etc. is such an engine, as comprises or consists of several lesser engines; and this compounded machine, in conjunction with the laws of motion, freely established and still maintained by God, among its parts, I look upon as a complex principle, whence results the settled order or course of things corporeal.[9]

Although one could visualize the human body (an organized aggregate of corpuscles) as a separate operative entity, it was in reality but a component of a larger dynamic whole—the corpuscular system of nature. Any interactions between the "system" of the human body and the "system" of nature took place physically and predictably in accordance with the original laws of matter and motion set forth by God in the original design. Since all qualities of bodies were fully explicable in terms of these laws, there was no need to postulate occult correspondences or spiritual causes to link the two systems. The Aristotelian notion that "natural appetites" compelled bodies to act one way rather than another was unnecessary. Nature's regularities were built into the design. The linkages between bodies were immediate, direct, and physical and capable of being understood wholly in terms of the corpuscular hypothesis. Although our senses may distinguish a variety of qualitative changes in bodies as they interact, Boyle felt that ultimately they would be found to be reducible to simple mechanical laws. Boyle makes this quite clear in a passage in *Origin of Forms and Qualities:*

> If we fancy any two of the bodies about us, as a stone, a metal, &c. to have nothing at all to do with any other body in the universe, it is not easy to conceive either how one can act upon the other, but by local motion (of the whole body or its corporeal effluvia); or how by motion it can do any more than put the parts of the other body into motion too, and thereby produce in them a change of situation and texture, or of some other of its mechanical affections: though this (passive) body being placed among other bodies in a world constituted as ours now is, and being brought to act upon the most curiously contrived sensories of animals, may upon both these accounts exhibit many differing sensible phaenomena; which, however we look upon them as distinct qualities, are consequently but the effects of the often mentioned catholick affections of matter, and deducible from the size, shape, motion (or rest), posture, order, and the resulting texture of the insensible parts of bodies.[10]

This conception of how bodies interact within their environment had several important ramifications for medical investigation. In the first place, by postulating that matter in motion alone defines the state of a substance, Boyle required the medical investigator to have a good understanding of the various ways motion might be induced. The dynamics involved were to be conceptualized in corpuscular terms. It follows, then, that the physician should first have a general understanding of the corpuscular philosophy, for it is the basic model upon which he might build a rationale for medical decision making.

Boyle's idea of corpuscular interaction between the human body and its external environment also required that any discussion of the *uses* of any given part of the body consider the overall design of nature. As he stated, the "whole animal itself, the use of whose particular parts is under inquiry, is but a part of that greater body, the universe; and therefore cannot easily be supposed to have been framed and furnished with the parts it consists of, meerly for its own sake."[11] Thus one cannot say that a given part was made for some particular aspect of an animal's welfare without qualifying how this is consistent with the general design of nature as a whole.

Boyle's insistence that the macrocosm and the microcosm were both subject to the same laws of motion made it easier for him to draw analogies between observed activities in the world at large and operations taking place in the human body. Boyle believed that this type of analogical reasoning could be especially fruitful for an increased understanding of those changes of state or texture that could be identified as "disease." The correspondences between the human body and external nature that the Paracelsians had seen in terms of a spiritual identity, Boyle held to be due to an identity of *dynamics:*

> That the naturalist's knowledge may assist the physician to discover the nature and causes of several diseases, may appear by the light of this consideration, that tho divers Paracelsians (taught, as they tell us, by their master) do but erroneously suppose, that man is so properly a microcosm, that of all the sorts of creatures, whereof the macrocosm or universe is made up, he really consists; yet certain is it, that there are many productions, operations, and changes of things, which being as well to be met with in the great, as in the little world, and divers of them disclosing their natures more discernibly in the former, than in the latter; the knowledge of the nature of those things, as they are discoverable out of man's body, may well be supposed capable of illustrating many things in man's body, which receiving some modifications there from the nature of the subject they belong to, pass under the notion of the causes or the symptoms of diseases.[12]

Boyle's denial of a directive principle in nature made him reject the maxim "Nature always does what is best." Interactions between a body and its environment were not purposive but wholly neutral. Boyle also refused to employ the term "preternatural" in its common definition, since this implied a distinction between "correct" and "improper" natural activity. He much preferred that the terms "customary" and "non-customary" be used in describing interactions occurring in nature, since these terms were freer of value judgment.[13]

Boyle's view that the given state of a body was solely a manifestation of mechanical interaction of corpuscles determined how he defined health and disease. If adequate body functioning, or "health," was not considered the result of any intrinsic striving for self-preservation, then the state of health was no more than a "compound accident," a composite of several qualities that coexisted at a given point in time.[14] Health thus was defined in holistic terms as a fortuitous composite of the various separate textures of the parts of the body that resulted in the body's operating as an efficient system.

"Disease" was defined in similarly value-neutral terms, but here the composite of qualities was perceived as being unfortuitous for efficient operation of the system as a whole. In the diseased state, the texture of one or several of the body's parts had become altered in such a way as to alter the overall functioning of the body. Thus, Boyle viewed disease not as a distinct "entity" or malevolent force but as a physiological state. Boyle's definition of disease is, then, a "physiological" rather than an "ontological" one.[15] Disease was perceived as a *deviation* from a prior state in which the body had functioned adequately as an engine. The degree of deviation determined the severity of the disease; the effect of disease was manifested as disordered function.

Although Boyle defined the diseased state wholly in terms of physiological organization, his views on the *causes* of disease involved the postulation of physical "triggers" acting upon a given part of the body; therefore, his concept of disease causation can be termed "ontological."[16] The actions of these physical triggers are described in terms of the corpuscular hypothesis. A disease cause impinges upon a given part of the body to promote a textural change, which manifests itself as impaired function. That the locus of the disease cause is outside the affected body part, that is, in its external environment, follows from the principle of inertia, which holds that a body will maintain a given state until acted upon by something external to it.

The cause of disease was not considered to be inherently evil. It was simply a factor of material corpuscles' impinging on the body from outside, which affected the motions of the corpuscles within the body in such a way that efficient functioning of the body became impeded. The cause of disease did not act in response to a deleterious directive principle either external to it or intrinsic within it; it operated wholly in accordance with mechanical laws.

The Human Body and the Environment

The cause of disease could "act" in several different ways. In the most simple case, a trigger of disease (e.g., a poison) entered the body through ingestion, respiration, or by insinuation through pores of the skin, and its constituent corpuscles then acted directly upon a specific body part (whose pores were of a size suitable to admit them) to produce a malfunction. Furthermore, these corpuscles could move from part to part, causing sequential malfunctions (which were identifiable as progressive disease symptoms). Sometimes, however, the corpuscles of the cause of disease did not insinuate themselves within a specific part, but affected the overall dynamics of corpuscular movement in the body. Boyle suggested that this happened in the case of seasickness, the corpuscular movements defining the ship in motion being transferred to the body as a whole, producing "unwonted agitations" in it that only secondarily caused malfunction in a specific body part, such as the stomach.[17]

Boyle attempted to explain, as a corollary of this second case—when the mechanical motion of corpuscles is transferred to the body as a whole to alter its motion—that even passions can cause physiological alteration. He accepted the fact that certain emotions, such as grief or fear, can produce physiological effects. Passions, of course, arise in the mind, yet they too rely on the environment, since they are stimulated by real or imagined factors from the environment.[18] This process Boyle termed "supra-mechanical," which, one will recall, was the category of causation Boyle established to explain operations of nature that were consistent with its design—that is, operations that were not occult or arbitrary—but nonetheless not as yet explicable in formal mechanical terms. By such a "supra-mechanical" process, the passions became translated into the physical motion of corpuscles (located in the brain). From the brain, these agitated corpuscles traveled via the nerves to many other parts of the body, where they produced alterations of texture that were perceived as "symptoms."[19] By such logic, Boyle attempted to argue that physiological change in every case involves corpuscular interaction.

The corpuscular hypothesis provided a basic perceptual framework for explaining what was occurring in the body. The practical orientation of the physician, however, required that he focus on a less abstract level when conducting specific investigations. Boyle believed that the processes of change, even though ultimately referable to invisible corpuscular interactions, could be empirically investigated by noting the symptomatic effects. By direct observation of the patient, the physician could discover (and eventually predict) the course of the illness as the morbific matter metastasized through the body. Physiological changes might also be more fully understood through chemical analysis of body fluids. This would lead to practical discoveries that would provide insights into treatment and cure. Boyle felt that even general laboratory study of chemical processes, for example, fermentation, would eventually shed light both upon normal physiological activity and upon changes that resulted in disease.

Effluvial Action

Boyle made it clear that the physician must consider not only factors in the environment capable of gross observation by the unaided senses but imperceptible (yet still physical) factors as well. He suggested that a wide variety of small particles from the environment that were not immediately evident to the senses but potentially identifiable via chemical analysis could insinuate themselves into any material bodies to produce significant effects. These particles were themselves aggregates of corpuscles, each possessing qualitative characteristics determined by their particular corpuscular composition. He termed these "effluvia."

In the passage from *Origin of Forms and Qualities* cited above, Boyle maintained that a body in motion could act upon another body either in its entirety or by its "corporeal effluvia." Effluvia were invisible emanations, or "steams," that emitted from all gross bodies in nature. The idea of emanation per se was one of great antiquity, having its origins in the pre-Socratic concept of "pneuma" and the identification of soul and air.[20] The doctrine of emanations had undergone much development from the Greek period down to Boyle's time. Neoplatonists focused on the emanations of a universal soul, alchemists spoke of "spiritus" released when bodies were heated or dissolved, and atomists suggested that sense perception was due to infinitesimal material bodies that flowed off from substances to enter the appropriate pores of the ear or eye. Boyle, like the atomists, emphasized the material nature of effluvial emanations and explained their interactions in wholly mechanical terms. Investigation of effluvial composition became for him a plausible way of improving one's understanding of the specific causes of change in nature in general and, as we shall see, of particular causes of disease.

Aristotle had recognized two kinds of exhalations, terrestrial (called "fumes"), which were hot and dry, and aqueous (called "vapors"), which were hot and moist. Boyle felt that this categorization was overly simplistic, noting that "besides the greater and more simple masses of terrestrial and aqueous matter . . . there are very many mixed bodies that emit effluviums, which make, as it were, little atmospheres about divers of them." He added that "the steams of bodies may be almost as various as the bodies themselves that emit them; and that . . . we may . . . conceive them to have their distinct and determinate natures, oftentimes, tho not always suitable to that of the bodies from whence they proceed."[21] These various emitted effluvia were carried through the air and eventually insinuated themselves into other bodies whose pores were of an appropriate size and shape to receive them.

Boyle's arguments concerning the real existence of material effluvia and their tangible effects on the bodies they encountered are included in a large number of his published works, beginning as early as 1663 with his *Usefulness of Experimental Natural Philosophy,* in which he alluded to effluvia as a cause of disease. To his *Continuation of New Experiments Physico-mechanical touching the Spring and Weight of the Air,* published in 1669, Boyle appended "A Short Discourse of the Atmospheres of consistent Bodies; shewing, that even hard and solid Bodies (and some such, as one would scarce suspect) are capable of emitting Effluvia, and so of having Atmospheres." In his 1670 publication *Tracts about the Cosmical Qualities of Things,* Boyle discussed how effluvia in the air could produce various effects on bodies, including illness, giving special attention to effluvia emitted by substances deep in the earth. In *Origin and Virtues of Gems* (1672) he once again noted the presence of subterraneal effluvia, this time in his description of the formation of minerals, where the "virtues" of stones were seen to be the result of material effluvia combining with the substance of the mineral as it was forming.

Boyle's most thorough consideration of the existence of effluvia was presented in 1673, in his *Essays of the strange Subtilty, great Efficacy, determinate Nature of Effluviums.* The 1674 work *Suspicions about some Hidden Qualities of the Air* contains Boyle's conjectures concerning the ways in which effluvia could affect the composition of the air and their role as causal factors in pestilential diseases. In 1684 he published his *Experiments and Considerations about the Porosity of Bodies.* There he described how both animal and solid bodies contained pores (through which effluvia could be admitted). A year later, he dealt with the effects of the various effluvia contained in the air upon living bodies, specifically with regard to their effects on health, in "An Experimental Discourse of some Unheeded Causes of the Insalubrity and Salubrity of the Air." This treatise was an appendix to his *Essay of the Great Effects of Languid and Unheeded Local Motion,* a work in which he maintained that a great many changes could occur in a body as a result of effluvial activity, even though the motions involved were not grossly visible. The purpose of all these works was to establish that effluvia were real material entities, were extremely varied, and could produce significant physical effects.

Boyle took special pains to emphasize that even though they were often visible, effluvia were totally material. His *Essays of the strange Subtilty, great Efficacy, determinate Nature of Effluviums* were designed to argue for the existence of such finely material entities. It was most important for him to emphasize that the effluvial off-flow operated in a physical, not an occult, manner.

Effluvia could have many different qualities. Their properties, or "natures," were identical to those of the bodies emitting them.[22] Effluvia could have "magnetical" or "electrical" qualities and could be derived from animal, vegetable, mineral, or even celestial bodies.[23]

Despite the fineness of the matter of which they were composed, effluvia could exert significant physical effects. According to Boyle, effluvia could influence gross bodies (1) by their great number, (2) by their penetrating and pervasive nature, (3) by their celerity and other modifications of their motion, (4) by the congruity and incongruity of their bulk and shape to the pores of the bodies they acted upon, (5) by the motions they excited in the affected body, and (6) by the power of effectiveness (and extended range) provided them by the "catholic agents of the universe," by which he meant agents such as light, gravity, and the aerial atmosphere.[24]

Boyle maintained that effluvia could produce even more notable effects than grosser bodies:

> And indeed if we consider the subject attentively, we may observe, that tho it be true, that, caeteris paribus, the greatness of bodies doth, in most cases, contribute to that of their operation upon others, yet matter or body being, in its own precise nature, an unactive or moveless subject, one part of the mass acts upon another, but upon the account of its local motion, whose operations are facilitated and otherwise diversified by the shape, size, situation, and texture both of the agent and of the patient. And therefore, if corpuscles, tho very minute, be numerous enough, and having a competent degree of motion, even these small particles, especially if fitly shaped, when they chance to meet with a body, which the congruity of its texture disposes to admit them at its pores, and receive their either friendly or hostile impression, may perform such things in the patient, as visible and much grosser bodies, but less conveniently shaped and moved, would be utterly unable on the same body to effect.[25]

Despite their small size, effluvia could also produce notable effects if the body was continually exposed to them over a long period of time. Speaking of those types of effluvia that can cause disease, Boyle explained:

Though in a small compass of time the noxious Effluvia that rove in the Air, may be too thinly dispers'd in it, to insinuate themselves in any considerable number at the Pores of the Skin; yet, by reason of the continual contact of the Air (especially as to the Face, Hands, and some other parts) which may last day and night for many months, or perhaps years, there may be opportunity for a considerable number of morbifick Particles to insinuate themselves into the cutaneous Pores.[26]

Boyle defined the air itself as an aggregate of effluvia and the prime vehicle of effluvial transmission. This emphasis on air as a composite of separable substances rather than as elemental was a key point in Boyle's postulations concerning the effects of the environment upon individual bodies. Boyle categorized the air as containing three general types of particles:

The first is made of that numberless multitude . . . of particles, which, under the form of vapours or dry exhalations, ascend from the earth, water, minerals, vegetables, and animals, &c. . . . and diffuse themselves into the atmosphere. The second sort . . . consist of such exceeding minute parts, as make up the magnetical steams of our terrestrial globe, and the innumerable particles, that the sun and other stars . . . do either emit out of their own bodies, or by their pressure thrust against our eyes, and thereby produce what we call light. . . . [The third] sort of particles are those, which are permanently [elastical], and on that account may be stiled perennial air.[27]

Boyle is speaking here of atmospheric air, what he terms "air in its more vulgar and laxe signification," rather than "air . . . properly so called," by which he meant the "springy" corpuscles alone. Effluvia were not *of* the air but *in* it. Boyle explained that effluvial vapors rise and are carried by the air simply because their corpuscles are lighter than the "springy" corpuscles of perennial air.[28] Because of their lightness and small size, effluvia are able to insinuate themselves into pores of bodies where the larger "springy" air corpuscles cannot pass.[29] Boyle maintained that effluvia also could interact with each other while in the air, becoming changed chemically thereby. Furthermore, the air as a whole (composed of an aggregate of particles) could be considered as a menstruum, capable itself of altering bodies exposed to it.[30] Boyle was convinced that increased investigation of the composition of the air, which varied with time and place because of the ever-changing effluvial particles entering or leaving it, would explain many heretofore inexplicable events, especially phenomena commonly termed "action at a distance."

Given his long interest in the chemistry of minerals, Boyle was especially intrigued with effluvia originating from subterraneal substances. He appears to have shared the alchemist's notion that the earth's interior served as a kind of giant natural alchemical retort in which chemical reactions continuously took place, producing new substances and altering others. Boyle was convinced that a great number of "subterraneal menstruums" and "mineral juices" were at work within the earth and that their importance in the production of minerals had not yet been recognized. "It is not improbable," he said, "that there may be in the earth a much greater variety of minerals dissoluble by the subterraneal menstruums, and capable of concoagulation with petrescent juices, than authors have yet taken notice of: to which conjecture divers subterraneal productions, that I have met with, do strongly incline me. And from the number and various mixtures of these may proceed, not only a great variety of operative particles in precious stones, but a high degree of energy in some of them."[31]

Boyle argued that the earth had its own internal heat, which stimulated these various subterraneal chemical operations, much as the alchemist's furnace stimulated chemical operations in the laboratory. In his *History of Cold,* he attempted to provide empirical evidence of the earth's heat.[32] In "Of the Temperature of the Subterraneal Regions," he spoke of three temperature zones in mines: the uppermost, warmed by the sun, warm; the middle, cold; and the lowermost, hot. He suggests that the heat of this lowermost zone comes from an even lower region, still unexplored:

> It seems probable to me, that in these yet unpenetrated bowels of the earth there are great store-houses of either actual fires or places considerably hot, or (in some regions) of both, from which reconditories . . . or magazines of hypogeal heat, that quality is communicated, especially by subterraneal channels, clefts, fibres, or other conveyances, to the less deep parts of the earth, either by a propagation of heat through the substance of the fire or heat through the above-mentioned conveyances . . . or else by sending upwards hot exhalations and mineral steams, which by reason of the comparatively heavy minerals they consist of, and by reason of their being less dispersed nearer the places whence they proceed, are usually more plentiful in the deeper parts of the earth, and somewhat affect them with the quality that they brought from the work-houses where they were formed, and that they retain for some time after.[33]

Subterraneal effluvia were the vaporous products of these chemical operations in the earth's interior. These "steams" were sufficiently subtle and volatile to work their way up into the atmosphere (particularly through openings, such as cave entrances), there to be carried off with the air.

Boyle was by no means original in holding this view of subterraneal activity. The idea of substances growing and maturing in the womb of the earth was an ancient one. Aristotle himself had explained the formation of metals and minerals as a result of the congealing of vaporous and smoky exhalations deep in the earth.[34] In Boyle's time, however, the most interest in this notion was exhibited by the Paracelsians. Paracelsus had interpreted Creation itself as a chemical separation, and his followers applied this metaphor of chemical separation to a variety of natural events, particularly in explaining geological phenomena. Michael Sendivogius (1556–1636), a favorite iatrochemical author of Boyle's, suggested that distillations in the earth were the cause of mountain streams, while metals were the results of sublimations.[35] Johann Rudolph Glauber (1603–70), whose improvements on alchemical furnaces were much discussed by Hartlib and Boyle,[36] in 1658 used the analogy of the circulation of the blood to explain the growth and nourishment of metals in the earth, as well as the expulsion of "superfluities" by the "circulation" of salt water (the salts of which were considered to be a universal nutrient).[37]

What Boyle chose to emphasize was that activities deep inside the earth had hitherto unrecognized but extremely significant effects upon events on the surface. He drew attention to regional variations in the direction of the magnetic needle of a compass and suggested that subterraneal agents might be at work. Irregularities in atmospheric pressure, as measured by his barometers, could be explained, he believed, by local alterations in the air, which "proceed for the most part from subterraneal steams."[38] Boyle made particular note of mineral exhalations that affected the health of those individuals exposed to them. Like others in his day, he was cognizant of toxic fumes in mines and aware of the deleterious effects of volatile minerals such as arsenic, but he also suggested that "there may be other [mineral substances] endowed with medical qualities, and the exhalations of such minerals, either alone, or mixed with petrescent liquors, pervading duly-disposed earths, and bolusses, and other fluid, soft, or open substances, before their induration, may endow them with medicinal and other qualities."[39] According to Boyle, the presence in the air of these various types of mineral exhalations determined the relative salubrity or insalubrity of any given geographic region.[40]

Because a variety of subterraneal effluvia could be carried through the air, Boyle felt that further investigation would reveal that effluvial action could account for many phenomena heretofore attributed to "occult qualities." One might well argue that by postulating invisible effluvial interaction as the cause of various events, Boyle was simply substituting one abstraction for another; however, interpretations in terms of these invisible but material effluvia were consistent with, and thereby gave greater credence to, Boyle's overall corpuscular hypothesis. Such interpretations were an important goal for Boyle. Furthermore, by directing attention to the chemical identification and classification of various types of effluvia, Boyle hoped to encourage the physician to expand his understanding of the causes of specific diseases. Occult explanations did not lend themselves to further research; effluvial explanations did.

To illustrate the value to the physician of focusing on effluvial action, Boyle attempted to suggest the general mechanism by which effluvia could cause disease. He began by explaining that all bodies contained pores, which were defined as the interstices between corpuscles. Since the shape and size of corpuscles varied greatly, there was similarly great variety in the size and shape of the pores between them. Effluvial particles of a suitable shape and size could insinuate themselves into these pores to alter the dynamic relationship between the corpuscles of the body (or body part), thus causing a malfunction. Animal bodies, Boyle explained, were especially receptive to various effluvia (and other intrusions from outside the body) because the internal parts of such bodies were constantly kept moist by body fluids (which were themselves kept in motion by the vital heat). The moistness rendered animal bodies "more lax, and more penetrable by subtle spirits or other corpuscles."[41] Boyle held that effluvia entering through the pores of the skin could have even more immediate effects upon the body than could ingested substances, since the effluvia would gain more immediate entrance into the bloodstream.[42]

Although every type of effluvia that insinuated itself into pores of the body did not necessarily result in deleterious textural change, impairments of function (perceived as a diseased state) could occur as a result of some altered textures, for example, when the motion of body fluids was impeded because the usual conduits for fluid flow were "plugged up" or when changes to a solid body part as the result of effluvial intrusion rendered it incapable of performing its usual activity (such as processing nutrients).

Boyle emphasized that the effects of a single type of effluvia could differ depending on where in the body the effluvial particles lodged. Either the type of functions impaired or the degree of impairment could differ. This meant that a single agent (effluvial or other) could create a variety of symptoms within the body, a fact of which the physician should be made aware so that he would not wrongly categorize these different symptom patterns as different diseases when in fact they were but varying manifestations of the same disease:

I have long been prone to think that it is not necessary the number of specifically different morbific matters, (as physicians call actually noxious humours or other substances) in the human body should be near so great as that of the diseases it is obnoxious to; and consequently, that every disease, that has a distinct name assigned to it, does not always require a distinct sort of peccant matter to produce it; but that the same hurtful humour, or other agent, may produce sicknesses, that pass for different ones, (and accordingly have distinct denominations) only as the same morbific agent's bad effects are diversified, partly by its own greater or lesser quantity, and more or less active qualities, and partly (and indeed chiefly) by the particular natures, or structures and situations of the parts, that it invades.[43]

Boyle was convinced that specific types of effluvia could cause specific diseases and that through repeated observation the cause of disease could be identified. Identification would be easiest when observing the effects of substances whose chemical composition was especially toxic to man. The effluvial off-flow of such substances would be noticeably toxic as well. An example of this would be certain toxic effluvia found in mines. Inhaled and contact poisons were other examples. Because he knew the potency of mineral substances prepared in the laboratory, Boyle posited that the most toxic effluvia were those that arose from subterraneal regions. The chemical activity that occurred naturally in the earth's interior was quite varied, to the extent that new substances could be generated; the effluvial off-flow of these substances as they made their way into the atmosphere could produce effects on the body perceived as very unusual symptoms. Boyle used this explanation to argue that such subterraneal effluvia were the source of many of the diseases physicians in that period had identified as "new diseases": "Nor am I sure . . . that some subterraneal changes, or some yet unobserved commerce between the earth and other mundane globes, has not an interest in the origin, countenance, and expiring of these diseases that physicians call new, which invade whole countries (and sometimes greater portions of the earth) and last very many years, if not some ages, before they come to be extinct."[44]

Boyle asserted that "it is likely that divers epidemical diseases are, in great part, produced by subterraneal effluvia."[45] Epidemic disease posed one of the most pressing and recurrent problems for physicians of Boyle's day. Boyle had lived through the Great Plague of London of 1665 and had written a long moralistic discourse about it.[46] Explanations for the outbreak and spread of epidemic disease lacked experimental verification, and it was difficult to understand just why the plague would break out in one place and not another, especially if one regarded as causes of the plague traditional factors such as "intemperance of the air, especially in point of heat, stench of dead bodies killed in fights, unwholesomness of aliments, malevolent aspects of celestial bodies, high provocations of the divine justice."[47]

Boyle believed that his ideas on effluvial action, particularly with regard to subterraneal effluvia, offered a logical explanation for the regional outbreak and spread of plague as well as the varying severity of the epidemic between neighboring locales. He was convinced that "the ascending Corpuscles of those Mineral Bodies, being most of them solid and subtile, may produce in the Bloud; and so in the Body, far more odd, and violent Symtomes, than the peccant Humours that use to beget ordinary Diseases." Those physicians who sought the cause of the plague in manifest qualities of the air, such as intemperate heat, were wrong, for there was no discernible causal relationship between such manifest qualities and plague occurrences. The air was, however, the medium of transmission for effluvial particles, and Boyle therefore maintained that the plague was likely due to "Noxious Subterraneal Fumes . . . suddenly, and without any warning belch'd up into the Air [which] by depraving it, produce fatal Diseases in many of those that are constantly surrounded by it, and draw it in, almost every moment, with their breath."

The continuance of plague could be explained by the fact that effluvia could *propagate:* "I think it very possible that divers Subterraneal Bodies that emit Effluvia, may have in them a kind of propagative or self-multiplying power," Boyle stated. He suggested that this power (which he saw as chemical, not vitalistic) might be something analogous to fermentation or a ripening process. He also noted that minerals and "other fossiles" were so abundant and so crowded together that they could emit effluvia for a very long time without becoming depleted. The extent and direction of spread of the pestilence from the point at which these subterraneal fumes escaped into the atmosphere depended on the prevailing winds.

Boyle even speculated about what type of mineral exhalations might have produced some types of plague, basing his conjectures upon his own knowledge of chemical substances. He first suggested "orpiment," that is, trisulfide of arsenic, a compound found naturally:

> What these Mineral Substances are, whose steams produce such odd and dismal Symptomes, I think exceedingly hard to determine. Yet, if I were to name one sort, I should perhaps think the least unlikely to be Orpiment. For, of the Poysonous Minerals we are acquainted with, I know not any of which there is greater quantity in the Bowels of the Earth, especially taking

> that name, in the latitude allowed it, by those skilful men, that make three sorts of it, viz. Yellow, Red, and White Orpiment, divers of whose mischievous Effects seem to agree well enough with the Symptomes of some Plagues, and may be guessed to have at least a considerable interest in the production of them.

He went on to qualify this suggestion, however, maintaining that he did not mean orpiment in its pure form:

> But yet, to speak candidly, I do not think that these Minerals are the causes, even of all those Pestilences whose efficients may come from under the Ground: For several reasons, and some drawn from Experience, make me think that the Subterraneal Regions have many kinds of very mischievous fossiles, of which Physicians, and even Chymists, have no knowledge, and for which they have not any distinct names; and that the various associations of these, which Nature may by fire and menstruums make under Ground, and perhaps in the Air itself; may very much increase the number, and variety of hurtfull Matters, and also heighten their hostility to Humane Bodies: as I think may be argued from the factitious White Arsenick that is commonly sold in Shops, which tho usually made of Orpiment, by the addition of so innocent a body as common Salt (which is found in great plenty under Ground), is observ'd to be far more poysonous than Orpiment itself.

Boyle believed that subterraneal effluvia were a much more plausible cause of plague than the factors cited by traditional authorities. He felt that celestial causes were too indeterminate, climatic factors too inadequate, and attributions of plague to divine wrath too nonspecific to explain why plague would manifest itself in a particular geographic area. Effluvial interaction offered an interpretation consistent with his fundamental views of matter. He suggested that a study of subterraneal regions and of the chemical composition of the substances contained in various mineral deposits would ultimately prove profitable to physicians in their attempts to determine the causes of various diseases.

Investigation of Minerals and Mineral Waters

Boyle expanded his own general research on geological phenomena to include a specific consideration of the health-related aspects of minerals. The passages already cited from his *Origin and Virtues of Gems* are indicative of this medical interest. Although Boyle's initial motivation for investigating mineral resources probably stems from the practical Baconian program of developing comprehensive histories of a country's natural resources for the general increase of knowledge, any findings relevant to human health would have been specifically of interest to Boyle. Thus, when in 1664 Boyle accepted membership in the Company of Royal Mines, as Louis More points out, "he made many inspection trips, exploring the minerals and soils of the country, and their possible uses for both industrial and medicinal purposes."[48] Letters to Boyle from Samuel Colepresse, written during the years 1666–67, include much information concerning minerals. To one of these letters, dated 1 February 1666/67, is appended a list of ninety items entitled "Answers to the queries of the honourable Robert Boyle, touching mines in Devonshire and Cornwall."[49] Several of these items relate specifically to health, such as item 4, which reads, "Our inhabitants, especially in the most mineral places, are very healthy, and live commonly to a great age," and item 40, dealing with fatalities occurring from "sudden damps" in the tin mines.

Although many subterraneal airs were considered toxic, and although effluvial exhalations from the "bowels of the earth" were cited as the cause of epidemic diseases, Boyle held that living near mineral deposits could have healthful advantages, as the above comment regarding the longevity of inhabitants of "the most mineral places" indicates. The benefits of mineral spas were at that time very well known, and Boyle shared with many of his contemporaries an interest in investigating mineral waters in order to discern their chemical composition and explain their medical efficacy. An extensive literature on the subject of mineral waters had been amassed since Italian physicians of the Middle Ages first studied local springs to determine their medicinal value and wrote down their findings.[50] The analysis of mineral waters was taken up with some vigor by the Paracelsians of the sixteenth and seventeenth centuries, who developed a variety of chemical tests for aqueous solutions.[51]

The discovery of the mineral springs at Scarborough and Knaresborough in 1626 resulted in much renewed interest in England in the analysis of spa water. One account of the Scarborough spa, written by Robert Witty in 1660, initiated a debate over methods of analysis. Witty questioned the results of the oak gall test, which had been used since antiquity as the most common color indicator for testing the presence of iron or vitriols (metallic sulfates). In 1685 Boyle published a work entitled *Short Memoirs for the Natural Experimental History of Mineral Waters,* in which he sketched a general outline for a comprehensive "history" of mineral waters, focusing especially on analytical techniques and the investigation of medicinal effects. Boyle's comments reveal that he fully appreciated the difficulties involved in achieving a thorough analysis of the chemical composition of the various spa waters. Nonetheless, he suggested experimental refinements that would permit better determinations. Boyle included a long discussion on the proper use of the oak gall test, indicating how and to what extent it could be valuable to analysis. He enumerated other methods for ascertaining the chemical composition of mineral waters. Some of these, such as flame tests and identification of crystalline structure, were based on information gleaned from earlier authors, especially the Paracelsians.[52] Other analytical methods that he mentions he developed on his own, for example, the specific gravity test and the use of syrup of violets to detect alkalis. As a whole, Boyle's treatise played an important role in popularizing the various methods of solution analysis.

In addition to techniques for determining the chemical composition of spa waters, Boyle also suggested ways to determine empirically the medical efficacy of various mineral waters, taking into account such factors as which specific diseases warranted, and which proscribed, their use; what differences in effectiveness could be noted between waters drunk at the site of the spring itself and those drunk after being transported away in open or closed vessels; what dietary considerations should accompany their administration; how and in what dosages the waters should be administered; and what possible side effects could occur. He further recommended that "mechanico-medical trials" be made upon animals, such as injecting mineral waters into the veins of a dog, to determine their effects on the blood.[53]

Meteorological Interests

If knowledge of geological phenomena was important to an understanding of the impact of the environment on the human body, so was a knowledge of meteorological changes. Interest in the medical implications of climatic factors was not uncommon in Boyle's day, an age in which there appears to have been a dramatic revival of interest in Hippocratic notions identifying diseases with specific climatic conditions.[54] Comments on the relation of disease to the weather appear frequently in the diaries of Samuel Pepys, John Evelyn, and Jonathan Swift. Thomas Sydenham, the "English Hippocrates," went much further, attempting to correlate disease species with specific weather conditions.

Francis Bacon had encouraged the organized collection of information on the weather and had written, as one of his planned histories, *History of the Winds,* in which he forwarded queries concerning the origin, nature, and effects of atmospheric movements. Boyle's Oxford colleague Thomas Willis, in his treatise *On Feavers,* of 1659, saw in unseasonable atmospheric conditions the "procatarctic," or external common cause, of epidemic diseases.[55] Isbrand van Diemerbroeck, whose *De Peste* Boyle praised highly, carefully delineated the atmospheric conditions that he believed had prompted the 1636–37 plague epidemic in the Netherlands.[56]

Boyle investigated the subject of the weather and climate in several works, most notably in his *History of the Air.* He maintained that the positions, situations, and motions of celestial bodies played an important role in regulating general meteorological phenomena.[57] He maintained that regional atmospheric variations were due to the different types of effluvia carried in the air of different geographic areas or even in the same area over a period of time. Members of the same animal or vegetable species might differ in their characteristics depending on the climate in which they were found (a factor of importance to the experimenter utilizing such substances in his research).[58] Boyle also noted that "as the same kind of bodies may have differing qualities, and consequently uses in differing places; so they may have [differing qualities] if examined or employed at differing times, comprising under that name, together with the four seasons of the year, those peculiar seasons or periods of time, to which some signal change of qualities or state in particular bodies do belong."[59]

Boyle's focus centered on the chemical composition of the air and the changes in that composition that occurred when different effluvial particles commingled. He felt that observed atmospheric changes themselves were visible manifestations of chemical activity, writing in his *Essays of the . . . determinate Nature of Effluviums,*

> It might be worth while to consider, whether these coalitions of differing sorts of steams in the air, and the changes resulting thence of their particular precedent quantities, may not assist us to investigate the causes of divers sudden clouds and mists, and some other meteorological phaenomena, and also of divers changes that happen in the air, in reference to the coming in and ceasing of several either epidemical, or contagious diseases, and particularly the plague, that seem to depend upon some occult temperature and alterations of the air, which may be copiously impregnated by the differing subterraneal (not to add here, sidereal) effluviums, that not unfrequently ascend into it, or otherwise invade it, with pestiferous, or other morbifick corpuscles, and sometimes with others of a contrary nature, and sometimes too, perhaps, neither the one sort of steams, which may be supposed to have imbued the air, is in itself deleterious; nor the other salutary, but becomes so upon their casual coalition in the air.[60]

The Human Body and the Environment

Boyle was particularly fascinated by reports from travelers that in Cairo each June there occurred a sudden cessation of a plague that was endemic in that region. In both *Usefulness of Experimental Natural Philosophy* and *Essays of the . . . determinate Nature of Effluviums,* he cites the account of Prosper Alpinus, a physician who had lived and practiced medicine in Egypt. Alpinus noted the coincidence between the annual flooding of the Nile and the sudden cessation of the plague but concluded that the flooding was not the cause of the abating of the plague, attributing it rather to an "alteration of the air, produced by northerly winds, which then begin to blow."[61] This attribution of health-related changes in a region to the prevailing winds was a traditional Hippocratic interpretation.

Boyle, however, preferred an alternative explanation. He rejected the idea that the cessation of the Cairo plague and the flooding of the Nile was but coincidence, noting that Nile water contained a high concentration of niter (a fact that had been observed even by the ancients). Combining this fact with information from an English traveler, George Sandys, that upon the Nile flooding there is a "certain moistening emanation diffused throughout the air," Boyle suggested that "one might guess, that this strange phaenomenon [the cessation of the plague] may be chiefly occasioned by some nitrous, or other corpuscles, that accompany the overflowing Nile, and by associating themselves with what Hippocrates somewhere calls νοσερὰς ἀποῤῥοίας, disable them to produce their wonted pernicious effects." He emphasized that the effect could not be due to the increased humidity of the air alone, stating:

> That these sanative steams perform their effects merely because they are moist, I presume naturalists will scarce pretend; but . . . they may be of such a nature, as by their coalition with the morbifick corpuscles, to encrease their bulk and alter their figure, or precipitate them out of the air or clog their agility, or pervert their motions, and, in a word, destroy all, or some at least, of those mechanical affections, which made those corpuscles pestilential.[62]

Not only could effects on one's health be attributed to the chemical composition of atmospheric air but atmospheric pressure and air temperature could have an impact on the human body. In an entry in *Philosophical Transactions* for 24 February 1672/73, Boyle wrote:

> I am prone to suspect that the very alterations of the atmosphere, in point of weight, may, in some cases, have some not contemptible operations, even upon man's sickness or health; as when the ambient air, for instance, grows suddenly very much lighter than it was before, or than it was wont

> to be, the spirituous and aerial particles that are plentifully harboured in the mass of blood, will naturally swell that liquor, and so may distend the greater vessels, and not a little alter the celerity and manner of the circulation of the blood by the capillary arteries and veins.[63]

In *History of the Air,* Boyle notes that warm air affects the "blood, juices, and spirits" of the human body via the agitations produced by heat. He qualifies this statement, however, by noting that another effect of warm air is to solicit the emission of effluvia from diverse bodies (which could not emit such effluvia at colder temperatures) and that "these effluvia may be the true and immediate causes of divers effects, that are unwarily ascribed to the mere heat of the air."[64]

Changes in the moisture content of the air also could result in some alterations in the body (although, as we have seen, this factor alone was not specific enough to produce dramatic changes, such as mollifying the plague in Cairo). Humid conditions could relax the pores of the body, which would allow moist air particles to gain easier entry into the body, where they could be absorbed by internal body membranes and cause them to become bloated. Boyle maintained that moist air particles could even gain access into the pores of bones, distending them and "making the parts bear hard against one another (which they did not at all before) at the junctures or articulations."[65] In this case too, distended tissues would alter the efficient flow of fluids within the body.

Boyle encouraged detailed regional studies of atmospheric conditions, and particularly of the chemical composition of the air, which he felt could be aided by the use of instruments such as the weatherglass (thermometer), the barometer, and the hygroscope (which measured atmospheric humidity). He also suggested experiments to ascertain the effects of the air on certain substances. He felt that local weather diaries would prove particularly useful in revealing any unusual meteorological trends or patterns, and he urged investigators to compare data from widely dispersed areas. Ultimately, Boyle hoped that such data collection would yield practical results not only for medicine but for husbandry, gardening, and even "in our oeconomical or civil concerns."[66]

Boyle's *History of the Air* includes the results of some of his own research, accounts of the research of others, and data from a weather diary compiled by his friend John Locke at Oxford and London from June 1666 to June 1683.[67] Boyle initially had interested Locke in the collection of such information, and Locke, in turn, tried to encourage others, such as his acquaintances traveling to distant lands, to take instrument readings and keep weather diaries. Locke became particularly fascinated with this subject, even to the point of sending out questionnaires with Charles Goodall for the purpose of obtaining bills of mortality, information about disease, and weather observations for every part of the world.[68]

Summary

It is evident that in forming his ideas on environmental effects on health, Boyle borrowed much from earlier thought but extended it and placed it in a corpuscular framework. Hippocratic notions of the influence of climate and weather conditions on health are combined with Paracelsian notions of subterraneal chemical activity. What is of interest is the way Boyle utilized his corpuscular hypothesis to relate these concepts and develop a logically consistent model of dynamic interaction that could explain a wide variety of conditions causing altered function in the human body without recourse to occult principles. Because of his particular interest in the action of chemically distinct effluvia, Boyle blended qualitative considerations with mechanistic principles to derive hypotheses that gave new insights into disease and underscored the notion of the body as a physicochemical system. This particular perspective on the body as it existed in its external environment was to prove very useful to medicine, especially in later centuries as knowledge of both physiology and chemistry became more sophisticated. In Boyle's own day this vision served as a speculative, though intriguing, framework for investigating the impacts of environment on health.

Because he emphasized that the human body was a system affected at every moment by its environment, Boyle had to explain how the human body could retain its integrity at all. Traditional vitalistic notions of an inherent tendency toward self-preservation were clearly unacceptable in his materialist philosophy. How Boyle accounted for the tenacity of the body to sustain itself in the face of forces that acted to disturb it, while maintaining the logical consistency of his holistic model of corpuscular activity, is the subject of chapter 5.

CHAPTER FIVE

The Restoration of Health

Altering the Dynamics of the Body

Boyle's views on therapy, like his views on disease, were predicated on the idea that disorder was ultimately an alteration of the dynamic pattern (or "texture") of the body induced by external factors. By his reasoning, if a textural alteration in a certain body part caused the body mechanism to malfunction, the proper corrective was to restore the texture to its former pattern. The restoration of texture could be accomplished by promoting a change in the motions or substantive composition of the constituent corpuscles.

As noted earlier, this view owes much to the concept of inertia: the body as a viable, organized system of interacting components will maintain itself until something intrudes to alter the status quo; the altered state will continue until some other physical event occurs to cause a reconfiguration of texture. The primary goal of the physician was to restore the body to its prior "efficient" state of operation. It is essentially an equilibrium model, then, that underlies Boyle's conceptualization of disease and cure.

Unlike the traditional Galenic equilibrium model, in which therapy was directed toward achieving a proper balance of the four humors of the body, Boyle's more generalized model focused on altering the dynamics of the interactions occurring at the corpuscular level. Emphasis was placed on the motions within a system rather than on the quantity or quality of several specific humors. One way to restore the body to its former arrangement might, in fact, include altering the humoral components, but Boyle's model allowed for much broader strategies, such as prompting change by inducing localized chemical change via specific medicines.

The most common way to restore the body to its former pattern was to administer appropriate drugs. However, Boyle also suggested that emotional stimuli could alter intestine motions in such a way as to promote cure. For example, Boyle accepted the notion that sudden frights could cure acute fevers.[1] He also accepted the folk wisdom that victims of tarantula bites could be cured by certain music, to which he gave a physical (corpuscular) explanation:

> [The music] proves suitable to the particular nature of the patient's body, or that of the poison, producing there such a motion, or determination of some former motion of the spirits, or the humours or both, as by conducting the spirits into the nerves and muscles inservient to the motion of the limbs, doth make the patient leap and dance, till he have put himself into a sweat, that breathes out much of the virulent matter, which hath been probably fitted for expulsion, by some change wrought in its texture or motion, or those of the blood, by the musick.[2]

Boyle's primary contention was that the success of a given curative agent depended on its ability to affect the corpuscular interactions within the body.

> A living human body is not to be looked upon as a mere statue . . . but [as] an admirably framed engine, consisting of stable, liquid and pneumatic substances, so exquisitely adapted to their respective functions and uses, that oftentimes the effects of an agent upon it *are not to be measured so much by the power of that agent considered in itself, as by the effects that are consequently produced* by the action of the parts of the living engine itself upon one another.[3]

Since curative action takes place at the corpuscular level, a substance need not be of great quantity or even be itself visibly perceptible to be efficacious. The main requirement was that a change be prompted in corpuscular movement that would result in the body's recovering its former dynamic composition.

An important aspect of Boyle's conceptualization was that it was not always necessary for the physician to intervene, for several factors naturally prevented the changes in texture that might often lead to illness. In the first place, the body as an inertial system possessing a stable arrangement had, by virtue of its organization, the ability to maintain itself in the face of external forces so as not to be easily prone to disorder in the first place. Boyle explains, "In a human body the causes, that disorder it, are oftentimes but transient; whereas the structure of the body itself, and the causes, that conduce to the preservation of that structure, are more stable and durable, and on that account may enable the engine to out-last many things that are hostile to it."[4]

"Divulging of Useful Truths in Physick"

This ability was strictly a result of the relative stability of the dynamic composition of the body within its external environment; by no means was it due to any sentient force of self-preservation present in nature. The holistic integrity of the human body in nature was solely a factor of its design:

> I conceive . . . that the wise and beneficent Maker of the world and of man, intending, that men should, for the most part, live a considerable number of years, in a condition to act their part on the mundane stage; He was pleased to frame those living automata, human bodies, that, with the ordinary succours of reason, making use of their exquisite structure fitted for durableness, and of the friendly, tho undesigned, assistance of various bodies, among which they are placed, they may in many cases recover a state of health, if they chance to be put out of it by lesser accidents than those, that God, in compliance with the great ends of the general providence, did not think fit to secure them from, or enable them to surmount. Many things, therefore, that are commonly ascribed to nature, I think may be better ascribed to the mechanisms of the macrocosm and microcosm, I mean of the universe and the human body.

Providence alone ensured the body's ability to sustain itself (within limits) in its environment.

In the second place, even when the body malfunctioned, it was found often to be capable of correcting itself without external intervention. At the corpuscular level, this could be attributed to the motion of restitution (see above, chapter 2). On the visible level, this restorative motion was observed as the medical "crisis." In traditional humoral theory, Nature was the directive force orchestrating this event. Nature "sensed" the imbalance in the body and, seeking to preserve the body, initiated the cooking or ripening process by which humors became appropriately mixed and excess humors were made fit for evacuation. In the corpuscular view, crises occurred simply because of an elastical characteristic of the aggregate of corpuscles to move to a former, more stable state when disturbed. As Boyle explained, this characteristic was built into the design of nature:

> The universal opinion of physicians is, that it is that intelligent principle they call nature which, being solicitous for the welfare of the patient, and distressed by the quantity or hurtfulness of the morbific matter, watches her opportunity (especially when it is concocted) to expel it hastily out of the body, by the most safe and convenient ways which, in the present condition of the patient, can be taken: and I, on the other side, attribute crisises to the wisdom and ordinary providence of God, exerting itself by the

mechanism partly of that great machine the world, and partly of the smaller engine the human body, as it is constituted in the patient's present circumstance.

The evacuations prompted by the medical crisis were also interpreted in wholly mechanical terms:

> It will often happen that the fibres, or motive organs of the stomach, bowels, and other parts, being distended or vellicated by the plenty or acrimony of the peccant matter, will, by that irritation, be brought to contract themselves vigorously, and to throw out the matter, that offends the parts, either by the emunctories or common shores of the body, or by whatever passages the proscribed matter can be with more ease discharged.

Boyle brought forth empirical evidence to support his contention that the medical crisis is a purely mechanical reaction and not the result of a directive force. He noted that some crises are fatal or leave the patient in a worse condition than before; that crises are not precipitated in all diseases, even though some diseases in which they are not present are potentially fatal; and that some bodily reactions commonly interpreted as forms of crisis may occur shortly after death, when obviously there can be no design of saving the patient. Like any other reaction in nature, the medical crisis operates totally in accordance with the laws of matter and motion established by God. Since these laws were formulated to apply *generally,* with the purpose of preserving the whole of God's design, the crisis could not be interpreted as nature's means of protecting any single individual.

The Physician as Minister of Nature

In light of the body's mechanical ability to deal with malfunction, Boyle maintained that the physician should see his role as one of helping the body correct itself: "I think the physician . . . is to look upon his patient's body, as an engine, that is out of order, but yet is so constituted, that, by his concurrence with the endeavours, or rather tendencies, of the parts of the automaton itself, it may be brought to a better state."

In most cases this meant that the physician should act in tandem with the body's own mechanical tendencies:

> If therefore he find, that in the present disposition of the body there is a propensity or tendency to throw off the matter, that offends it, and (which ought to be some way or other expelled) in a convenient way, and at commodious places; he will then act so, as to comply with, and further, that way of discharge, rather than another; as, if there be a great appearance,

> that a disease will quickly have a crisis by sweat; he will rather further it by covering the patient with warm cloaths and giving sudorific medicines, than by endeavouring to carry off the peccant matter by purging or vomiting, unseasonably hinder a discharge, that probably will be beneficial.

If, however, the physician determined that the body's normative mechanical responses would exacerbate the patient's condition, he could intervene to temper these responses.

> Thus, tho nature in dropsies importunately crave store of drink, the physician thinks himself obliged to deny it; as he does what they greedily desire, to his patients of . . . that distemper they call pica, though the absurd and hurtful things, as very unripe fruit, lime, coals, and other incongruous things, be earnestly longed for. Thus also the chirurgeon does often hinder nature from closing up the lips of a wound, as she would unskilfully do, before it be well and securely healed at the bottom. So the physician does often, by purging or phlebotomy, carry off that matter, that nature would more dangerously throw into the lungs, and expel by frequent and violent coughs.

The physician, in essence, should be nature's "minister":

> I look upon a good physician, not so properly as a servant to nature, as one, that is a counsellor and friendly assistant, who, in his patient's body, furthers those motions and other things, that he judges conducive to the welfare and recovery of it; but as to those, that he perceives likely to be hurtful, either by increasing the disease, or otherwise endangering the patient, he thinks it is his part to oppose or hinder, though nature do manifestly enough seem to endeavour the exercising or carrying on those hurtful motions.

Since nature acts mechanically, the physician is permitted to be interventive and to use his own judgment, based on his knowledge of the patient's overall situation. Allowing physicians this freedom of action makes it even more crucial that they have a broad understanding of both the patient and the external environment, that is, an insight into the design and functioning of nature, so that they can make informed medical decisions.

Even though he is free to intervene, the physician should use the most gentle remedies available to achieve the desired effects without weakening the body or interfering with the body's own restorative mechanisms (when these are deemed safe). For example, Boyle felt that remedies given for the sole purpose of prompting quick physical evacuations were to be recommended only in dangerous cases where the natural evacuation process would prove deleterious. Remedies that worked chemically to transform the morbific matter itself were more effective. This emphasis on moderate, calculated interference by a physician who understood how the body responded to malfunctions is central to Boyle's therapeutic methodology.

Explanations of Drug Action

Because of Boyle's ontological view of the causes of disease and his interest in the possibility of prompting change of texture via chemical alteration of the matter of the body itself, he was particularly interested in "specifics," that is, drugs targeted to a single disease, as opposed to general evacuatives or elixirs, given for a wide spectrum of ailments. In his treatise *Of the Reconcileableness of Specific Medicines to the Corpuscular Philosophy,* Boyle set down his arguments for preferring specifics and provided a feasible explanation for their action on the basis of the corpuscular hypothesis. He noted the various ways in which specifics may be curative: (1) by "resolving" certain types of morbific matter, making it fit for expulsion; (2) by "mortifying" the overacidity of particles infesting the mass of the blood, which cause undue coagulations (these coagulations, of course, impeded motion); (3) by precipitating peccant matter out of the fluid parts of the body; (4) by strengthening the heart or other organs (so that the body's own resources would become strong enough to counter the illness); (5) by producing in the blood such motions as to allow it to correct or expel the morbific matter or other cause of disease; (6) by "neutralizing" the peccant matter so that it becomes harmless even if not expelled.

Boyle considered specifics to be especially effective in cases of chronic disease.

> It is known that many diseases, and those oftentimes stubborn and chronical, proceed from certain tough or viscous humours, that obstruct the passages, whereby the blood should circulate, or other useful liquors be transmitted; and these peccant humours are oftentimes so viscid and obstinate, that ordinary remedies will do little or no good upon them. And yet a specific may, by the smallness and congruous figure of some of its corpuscles, get through the pores into the recesses of this stubborn matter: and by their solidity, figure, and agitation, promoted by the heat of the patient's body, may dissolve and ruin the texture of the morbific matter, and render it capable of being proscribed by nature. . . . Thus the blood, or some other liquor of the body, being (to use the chymist's phrase) impregnated with the friendly and operative particles of the remedy, becomes an appropriated menstruum in reference to the peccant matter.[5]

Boyle believed that specifics had advantages over traditional galenicals, which were usually compound drugs prepared so as to achieve that precise degree of hotness, coldness, wetness, or dryness needed to restore the humors in the body as a whole to a healthy state of (qualitative) balance. While Boyle did not deny that galenicals could be efficacious in affecting evacuations and strengthening depleted humors or that they were sometimes cheaper and more easily obtained than were many specific drugs (which usually required chemical preparation), he maintained that specifics were less traumatic; more appropriate, since they could be tailored to affect only certain types of physical matter in the body; and often more immediately efficacious than traditional galenical remedies.[6]

Boyle held that a specific drug useful in curing one given disease would not necessarily cure another disease considered akin to it, "for the presumed cognition may not be so great, but that some dissimilitude of texture in the morbific matters may make one of them unfit to be wrought upon by the same menstruum, that dissolves the other."[7] Furthermore, specific medicines might sometimes fail because of individual variations in the body constitutions of different patients.

For these reasons, Boyle was skeptical that any "universal remedy" could be discovered that would cure all diseases. Rather, he suggested that when a certain drug was deemed efficacious in alleviating a wide variety of ills, its success was probably due to the fact that all these symptoms, though perceived as separate diseases, were actually due to a single disease cause manifesting itself differently in different organs. The drug worked because it traveled through the bloodstream to interact chemically with the specific morbific corpuscles.[8]

A basic problem for those attempting to describe the action of specifics was to explain how such drugs could resist becoming chemically altered in the course of their transit through the body. Boyle admitted that a drug substance could be altered once it entered the body. He particularly cautioned that the same drug could have different effects depending on whether it was ingested or externally applied. He noted as well that drug efficacy depended upon the time spent in transit and the patient's current condition. These variables had to be considered in any thorough study of the efficacy of specific medicines.

Boyle utilized the basic premises of corpuscular interaction, however, to argue that it was possible for a drug to retain its chemical integrity even within the body, asserting that since the corpuscles of the drug would be fit to interact only with corpuscles of a suitable size and shape, the "texture" of the drug might remain unchanged until the drug was brought into proximity with these suitably shaped corpuscles. Thus it was possible for a drug to be transported essentially unaltered to the disease locus. This view is consistent with Boyle's arguments for the ability of the human body to maintain its integrity vis-à-vis the external environment. Only if a textural change was accomplished through physical contact at the corpuscular level could the body be distorted from its prior state.

Even if the specific drug interacted with corpuscles other than those in the part for which it was intended, the result of this interaction was not always unprofitable. For example, the blood, by reacting with the specific drug substance, could itself be turned into a menstruum, thus acquiring a curative ability of its own. Also, the specific drug, as the result of being acted upon, might be broken down in such a way as to become more easily assimilated at the disease locus.

> The remedy thus admitted into the mass of blood may, in its passage through the strainers [by which he means the liver, spleen, kidneys, and what he terms "local ferments residing in particular parts"], be so altered, either by leaving some of its parts there, or by having them altered by the . . . ferments, or by being associated with some other corpuscles, it may meet with in its passage; whereby the size, or figure, or motion of its small parts may be changed; or in a word, it may . . . receive so great an alteration, in reference either to some or other of the strainers, or other firmer parts of the body, or to the distempered blood, or some other fluid and peccant matter, that it needs not seem impossible, that by that time the medicine (crumbled as it were in minute corpuscles) arrives at the part or humour to be wrought upon, it may have a notable operation there. . . . And the same sanative corpuscles may perchance be also fitted to stick to, and thereby to strengthen such fibres of the strainers, or such other firmer parts of the body, as may need congruous corpuscles to fill up their little unsupplied cavities.[9]

Boyle did admit that drugs that had to pass through the digestive system were likely to be so broken down that they could lose their efficacy. Therefore, he emphasized the greater effectiveness of externally applied specifics, whose effluvia entered through the pores of the body and were immediately absorbed into the bloodstream, as these were less likely to be modified than drugs that were ingested. Boyle also believed that drugs that worked by effluvial emanation were especially useful as specifics because they could work effectively in quantities too small to weaken the body or contravene the body's own restorative mechanisms.

Boyle's belief in the power of effluvial action enabled him to provide a rational explanation for medical remedies that until then had been considered occult (and therefore outside the province of Galenic pharmacology), such as amulets or the weapon salve. He used similar reasoning to explain the surprising cures of the "Irish Stroker," Valentine Greatrakes, whose healing powers, which essentially involved touching the patient and "stroking out" the illness, became the sensation of London in the mid-1660s.[10]

Boyle held that Greatrakes transmitted from his body to that of the patient a material substance that acted as a specific drug to mollify the disease. Boyle anticipated the obvious objection to this hypothesis, namely, that Greatrakes claimed to cure a wide variety of diseases and that this would be beyond the power of a single specific drug. In answer, Boyle asserted that some specifics have a more extensive range of efficacy than others, citing the ability of certain spa waters to alleviate a wide variety of illnesses. He also reiterated that physicians might often diagnose as different diseases illnesses caused by a single morbific matter manifesting itself as different symptoms in different parts of the body.

Another explanation he gave for Greatrakes's cures was that the strong passions elicited in the patient during the dramatic healing performances might produce a commotion in the body sufficient to cause an alteration of its texture.[11] Recoveries achievable in this way would be due to the fact that the enhanced motion within the body allowed for speedier evacuation of the morbific matter. Such recoveries, however, could only account for some of Greatrakes's many documented cures. Boyle still thought it most plausible that something material was transferred from Greatrakes into the patient's body. Therefore, Boyle favored the notion that Greatrakes imparted some specific effluvia in the course of his contact with the patient. (Boyle was later to "test" this theory when, on one of the more than sixty occasions in which he directly witnessed Greatrakes's performances, he took over a curative procedure Greatrakes had begun, by stroking the patient himself with the inside of Greatrakes's glove, and noted that the patient reported himself cured.)[12]

Boyle insisted that whether Greatrakes efficacy as a healer was due to promoting commotions of the body's corpuscles or to introducing a curative effluvial substance, his cures could be explained fully in physical terms, and there was nothing miraculous or occult about his activities. A set of queries he set forth in a letter to Henry Stubbe includes, among many others, the suggestion that the chemical composition of Greatrakes's body fluids be determined.[13] Boyle urged his colleagues to observe Greatrakes's performances and provide written testimony on cures they had witnessed. He may also have inspired his friend Henry Oldenburg to speculate regarding the role of friction in his curing performances.[14]

Boyle must have recognized that Greatrakes provided him an excellent opportunity to display the value of corpuscular interpretations to explain seemingly occult phenomena. A great many of the most respected virtuosi of London were aware of Greatrakes's activities—his cures being the talk of the coffeehouses—and had pondered the cause of his powers. The unusual degree of success attributed to Greatrakes's faith healing made many feel compelled to explain his achievements, since he could not easily be dismissed as a fraud. Furthermore, Greatrakes had arrived on the London scene at a time of particularly intense debate between those who accounted for natural phenomena in terms of "plastic powers of nature" or other sentient or occult principles and those who preferred a mechanistic and materialistic view. Greatrakes thus became a kind of cause célèbre, both sides claiming that his curative powers supported their position. In fact, such arguments became so intensive as to result in a pamphlet war in the year 1666. It is in this context that Boyle's great interest in describing the physical and mechanical basis of Greatrakes's cures should be understood. Here was a case that profitably could be investigated along the lines Boyle had set forth for collaborative empirical research in general.

Boyle held that the best way to ascertain the efficacy of any curative agent was through empirical trials. He had always maintained that repeated research into the chemical nature of substances thought to be curative would greatly enhance the physician's knowledge. Boyle felt that chemical trials were necessary to determine the chemical composition and efficacy of all drug substances. Although he was particularly interested in discovering and describing drugs that acted as specifics, and especially those that appeared to operate by means of effluvial emanation, he believed that even well-known galenicals that had been in use for centuries could be better utilized if they were subjected to chemical analysis and their physiological effects were reinterpreted in terms of the corpuscular hypothesis.

A substance should not be rejected as inefficacious, Boyle urged, if it was observed to work successfully only part of the time. All known and accepted drugs had limitations; none were universally effective in all patients under all conditions. Of all areas of scientific inquiry, that of medical experimentation was the most difficult. Because of the complexity of the human body, as well as the inability to artificially reproduce conditions in the laboratory under which the number of variables could be controlled, exact experiments were impossible. A drug could have quite different effects on individuals of different constitutions. Furthermore, the composition of drugs used in the testing could vary considerably: drugs procured from apothecary shops were often adulterated, and even a drug properly prepared or procured could work differently depending on its age or even the time of year in which its ingredients were harvested. Despite the profound difficulties, Boyle held out the hope that by repeated trials, fairly conducted, investigators could obtain sufficient information to judge the efficacy of various remedies.

Boyle brought his extensive understanding of chemical activity and his technical skill to bear on his own efforts to ascertain the properties of drugs. For example, his prior knowledge of the characteristics of gold caused him to question whether one should regard potable gold as a remedy. He argued that since gold requires such a "very subtile liquor to volatilize it," the average chemical physician would never succeed in preparing true potable gold. If the resultant concoction was efficacious, as many had claimed, it could not be due solely to the properties of the gold. "If this or other preparations of *aurum potabile* prove good medicines, it would be farther inquired, whether the virtues may not in great part be rather attributed to the menstruum, than the gold . . . or to the association of the corpuscles of the gold, with the saline particles of the menstruum, into a new concrete, differing enough from gold, though never so well opened."[15]

Boyle believed that basic chemical skill was valuable in making determinations of the composition of drugs sold as secret remedies (usually at a high price), which were too compounded or disguised by their preparation to be identified by traditional nonchemical methods, such as tasting or smelling.[16] Also, one trained in the chemical art could investigate how mineral substances used only sparingly by physicians because of their potency might be made safer.[17] Boyle was convinced that the chemically trained natural philosopher could greatly extend the pharmacopoeia. The trials were time-consuming, the subject vast, and the research often required a high degree of chemical skill. Nonetheless, the natural philosopher who had such abilities could advance the physician's art considerably. Boyle insisted that a chemical perspective was essential:

> I have made several trials that have, I confess, much inclined me to think, that the fault is rather in us, than either in nature or chymistry that men do not, by the help of chymical experiments, discover more of the nature of divers medicaments, than hitherto they seem to have so much as aimed at. For though the abstruse endowments of specificks will not, I fear, be learned in haste, otherwise than by particular trials, and observations; yet many simples have other qualities, which seem chiefly to reside, though not in an elementary salt or sulphur, yet in a part of the matter that seems of kin to a salt or sulphur; such as sourness, saltness, a caustic or healing faculty, abstersiveness, and the like, upon whose account such remedies

> seem chiefly to work in a multitude of cases. And towards the investigation of such qualities, a chymist may oftentimes do much, without making all his trials in human bodies.[18]

Philanthropic considerations also motivated much of Boyle's personal research and writing about drugs. This is not surprising, since social welfare was the goal that underlay his scientific endeavor. His "Epistolical Discourse of Philaretus to Empericus, inviting all true lovers of Vertue and Mankind, to a free and generous Communication of their Secrets and Receipts in Physick," which called for increased access to recipes, certainly reflects this concern. There is further evidence of this goal seen in his *Medical Experiments,* a collection of recipes for simple and inexpensive medicinals that could be used by country people who had little access to more sophisticated medicine. Boyle selected for this compendium remedies that the general populace could easily prepare and whose ingredients were easily procurable. Because this work had a wholly practical aim, Boyle included in it empirical remedies whose efficacy had not yet been explained by any known formal theory. The criterion for inclusion of any remedy in this treatise was simply that credible witnesses had testified as to its efficacy.

Boyle insisted that all remedies be judged in a wholly unbiased manner. Drugs discovered by the unlettered empiric might prove as valuable as those discovered by the trained physician. He cautioned, however, that one should not put too much trust in empirics as medical practitioners, and he urged that if a person not trained in medicine had developed a successful remedy for one disease, that individual's medical practice should be limited only to treatment of that disease.[19]

The expense or rarity of the ingredients used was not, Boyle insisted, a valid determinant of a drug's efficacy. This was a point well taken in an age when considerable profit could be made off the gullible by insisting that the only appropriate remedy was an expensive one concocted of precious minerals, including "leaf-gold," rubies, and emeralds.[20] Although many of his chemist associates insisted that the newer iatrochemical remedies were far superior to traditional galenicals, Boyle refused to assume that this was universally true, preferring to qualify his position as follows:

> I love to look upon both chymical and Galenical remedies with an impartial eye, and think, that neither the former ought to be despised for the latter, nor the latter for the former: for as chymical remedies have commonly the advantages of being more durable, less clogging by their quantity, and less nauseated by patients; so Galenical remedies have, *when they are of equal efficacy,* the advantages of being more cheap, (at least quantity for

> quantity), more procurable, and sooner prepared. And such is the variety of cases arising from the variety of constitutions and distempers, that in some of them the former sort of remedies may be more proper, and in others, the latter may seem requisite; and in some also, both sorts may alternately be so useful, that neither of them can well be spared.[21]

Only by repeated trials could the relative efficacy of such drugs be determined.

Boyle preferred to work with simples rather than compound drugs for the obvious reason that simples were easier to analyze and therefore afforded precise information that could then be used to extend the *materia medica.*[22] Further, he felt that simples had distinct therapeutic advantages over compound drugs, and not only because they were usually cheaper. Rather than enhancing a remedy, polypharmacy actually could be counterproductive:

> I think it . . . not unreasonable to suspect, that, where a great many ingredients are blended into one medicine, one or other of them may have other operations, besides that designed by the physician: it may awaken some sleeping ferments, and if not produce a new distemper, may excite and actuate some other hostile matter, that lay quiet in the body before, and perhaps would have been little by little subdued by nature, if it had not been unseasonably roused and assisted by some ingredient, that perhaps was needlessly put into the medicine. I have had so many unwelcome proofs of this in myself, that it engages me to be the more careful to caution others against the like inconvenience.[23]

Boyle also noted that simples usually provided a greater dose of an ingredient than did compounds in which many ingredients were mixed. To those who objected that a simple would never be powerful enough to cure a disease that manifested itself by several differing symptoms, Boyle stated that since different symptoms may all be due to the same single morbific matter, a simple drug might well prove sufficient. In addition, a given simple could itself possess varied qualities that made it capable of having varied effects in the body. "In a simple medicine nature herself does oftentimes so well play the apothecary, as to render the compositions made in his shop unnecessary. For though we are wont to look upon this or that plant or mineral, as an entire and simple body, yet we may much mistake, if we look upon it as a homogeneous one."[24] Chemical trials, of course, would help reveal the variety of qualities of these simple substances.

An unconventional but promising new area for pharmaceutical investigation was that of substances known to be poisonous. Boyle was very interested in this subject, even though he felt the need to suppress publication of an early treatise he wrote entitled "Essay of Turning Poisons into Medicines," either because he feared that unscrupulous people might exploit this information for evil purposes or because, as Marie Boas Hall has maintained, the work lacks originality.[25]

Boyle felt that success in mollifying such powerful substances for medical purposes would be a great human achievement. The Paracelsians had also been inspired by the idea that poisons could be altered to produce exceptional medicines,[26] and their work was the starting point for Boyle's own investigations. Boyle noted in *Usefulness of Experimental Natural Philosophy* that God had so designed nature that "many poisonous bodies contain their own antidotes."[27] He expressed a similar sentiment in a later work where he wrote of a seemingly successful plague remedy containing arsenic used by a physician during the Great Plague of London in 1665: "If this [remedy] prove as successfull in other Plagues, as it did to those that us'd it in that of London; there will be just cause to admire and praise the benignity of Divine Providence, which in a poisonous Mineral, that probably does oftentimes concur to produce the Plague, has laid up a remedy for it."[28]

Boyle's "Essay of Turning Poisons into Medicine" is divided into three parts, dealing in turn with mineral, animal, and vegetable poisons.[29] While this work is by no means original, it does blend the work of others with his own commentary. Boyle suggests chemical procedures for rendering each poison harmless and gives specific recommendations for its use. For example, he relates that "by a few sudden detonations with saltpetre," antimony could be rendered white and innocent and would lose its vomitive quality. While its emetic properties would be removed, however, it still would contain other cathartic qualities that would allow it to be of use in purifying the blood. The mollified poison could also impede putrefaction. Boyle suggested ways to combine both antimony and mercury (a poison in its own right) and maintained that the resultant compound could be efficacious in diseases where all other medicines were completely useless. He emphasized that great caution should be exercised in using this medication because "it often works so violently, that tis as likely to take away the patient as the disease." Therefore, it was to be administered only as a last resort. (Boyle warned that apothecary shops often sold this preparation in adulterated form, and he provided information on how the drug could be prepared at home, using a recipe of Glauber's.)

Besides antimony, the section on mineral poisons focuses especially on mercury and arsenic. In the section on poisonous animals, Boyle concentrates on scorpions, spiders, and vipers (noting for the latter that he questioned whether vipers should, in fact, be classified as poisonous, since they acquired poisonous qualities only when enraged). In the section on vegetable poisons, he discusses only opiate preparations, concentrating his remarks on opiate laudanum.

Boyle's most original contribution to pharmacology is provided in a short treatise the full title of which is *Medicina Hydrostatica: Or Hydrostatics applied to the Materia Medica, Shewing How, by the weight that divers Bodies used in Physic have in Water, one may discover, whether they be genuine or adulterate.*[30] This work was published in 1690. Boyle tells us that he deliberately chose the running title *Medicina Hydrostatica* to parallel the title of an equally short treatise by the Italian experimenter Sanctorio Sanctorius, *Medicina Statica,* which described the use of the balance in the medical art.[31] In his treatise Boyle developed a method of weighing substances to compare their specific gravities and suggested that this method be used to test drug purity. Boyle had already advocated such specific gravity testing in the analysis of mineral waters. Here he advocated its general use in pharmacy. In his preface to the work, Boyle expressed the hope that this treatise would achieve a desirable effect, "by exciting the more curious among physicians, chemists, and others, to enlarge their inquiries; and by helping them to remark divers things relating to medicinal bodies, that they are wont to overlook."[32]

This statement of his intentions could be applied equally well to all of Boyle's research and writing on the subject of therapeutics. Since the human body existed in an environment that was the source of both potential maladjustment and potential cure, the broadest perspective that could be brought to bear on how the body reacted to external elements was the most instructive. To achieve this broadened vision, the physician needed an open mind and a willingness to utilize the expertise of others, even those not specifically trained in medicine. The body, after all, was not substantively different from other materially organized systems in nature. All obeyed the same general natural laws. Therefore, any learned individual could contribute to the quest for new ways of restoring health.

CHAPTER SIX

Boyle's Medical Thought in Its Contemporary Context

Boyle's interest in the subject of human health appears to have been motivated by religious ideals and a commitment to human welfare shared by others of his generation who sought to reform society. By embracing the idea of placing medicine under the umbrella of the new science, Boyle also reflects the intentions of other virtuosi, a number of whom had had medical training. True to his belief in the value of cooperative research, Boyle often extended the work of his close colleagues. His work at Oxford and later at the Royal Society especially reveals how much his own research reflects the predominant scientific problems under study by his circle of associates.

Boyle also gained recognition as a facilitator and popularizer of science. His everyday work often involved the validation and clarification of the ideas of his contemporaries. He became a respected figure, patiently tolerating an almost constant stream of visitors seeking his opinion or desiring demonstrations of novel experiments. Both in public and private life Boyle worked to disseminate new scientific hypotheses and empirical findings. His support was eagerly sought and valued by scientific researchers in England.

Reacting against the divisiveness in the medical community of his day, Boyle espoused an eclectic, open-minded, empirical approach, which he felt would best promote the goal of medical reform. Like many of his English compatriots, he used as his starting point for understanding physiology the work of William Harvey, with its focus on the activity of body fluids and the concept of the body as a hydraulic system. Fusing his chemical ideas to his corpuscular philosophy, he attempted to create a qualitative, comprehensive vision of how the human body operated in the context of its environment.

Despite Boyle's legendary disorganized way of working and the fact that his medical ideas came to be published in scattered fashion throughout his works, there is remarkable consistency in his medical thought.[1] At one time or another, he took up most of the topics important to physicians of his day and provided, by means of his corpuscular hypothesis, interpretations that together form a logical whole for understanding the human body in health and disease. The ideas he forwarded not only suggested an alternative theoretical framework for medicine but also had ramifications for medical practice, for example, with regard to the proper role of the physician and the degree and type of medical intervention appropriate in treating disease.

Boyle and the *Methodus Medendi*

Boyle and others in his day were motivated to ponder medical matters at such length because of the current crisis in the medical profession, fueled in part by increasing competition among practitioners but also by new perspectives toward nature that undermined traditional rationales for treatment. New empirical findings and methodological ideas strongly competed with older theories and methods. The established framework of Galen was being questioned, and this caused doubt to be cast upon time-honored Galenic rationales for treatment and, indeed, upon the basis for medical professionalism itself.

For the professional physician, this intellectual crisis caused as much confusion as did the threat that the proliferation of unlicensed practitioners would run the professional out of business. Since the High Middle Ages, the professional credibility of physicians had been linked to book learning and the ability to justify decisions by reference to an established view of how the human body functioned. But now, given competing philosophies and perceived deficiencies in the Galenic corpus, there was no longer a clear-cut referent by which professionals could be identified. Additionally, the successes of the new science in promoting the idea that nature was ultimately reducible to simple, regular laws caused many to wish that medicine too could be perceived as a rigorous scientific discipline. The need among learned physicians for a revised *methodus medendi* on which they could generally agree was great, if for no other reason than to ensure their professional integrity.

The traditional *methodus medendi,* which had been founded on Galen's essentially observational approach but had become calcified over time, now appeared dogmatic and even dangerous to medicine. The established *methodus medendi* was under tremendous challenge in Boyle's time, being attacked particularly by iatrochemists, who disputed Galen's functional view of disease and his predominantly evacuative therapy. In an analysis of the changes in the *methodus medendi* taking place in the sixteenth and seventeenth centuries, Jeffrey Boss has pointed out that Galen's method (as it was interpreted in this age) was vulnerable because, although it could be used to generate new knowledge, the method itself could not be an object of change and still maintain its utility.[2]

Even Boyle argued that the traditional *methodus medendi* encouraged unsafe practices by being overly deterministic and inflexible and that its classificatory constructs were too static and insufficiently heuristic. In an essay fragment contained in one of Boyle's notebooks held by the Royal Society of London, Boyle argues why one should not adhere blindly to the old *methodus medendi.* He first notes that "there is scarce any thing that has so much confin'd the generality of Physicians to the vulgar method of physick, and kept them from impartially considering the reasons and the practices of those that dissent from it, as the persuasion they have that the received method is most safe and any that deviate from it dangerous." Looking into this "persuasion," however, Boyle finds that physicians have no good reason to believe their traditional method safest, except "that it has been generally practised for many Ages, and that even by eminently learned as well as by ordinary Physicians." To this argument Boyle replies, "I frankly confess this were a weighty Argument, if every method of curing a Disease that has been imployed long and generally had been also imployed successfully." He notes, however, that "on the contrary it appears that it has been oftentimes unable to cure the Patients and diverse times has made them worse than it found them."[3]

Boyle also criticized the traditional *methodus medendi* for the excessive generality of its therapeutic precepts:

> The main thing that induces me to question the safeness of the vulgar *methodus medendi* in many cases is the consideration of the nature of those Helps they usually employ, and some of which are honored with the title of *Generous Remedies.* These helps are Bleeding, Vomiting, Purging, Sweating, and Spitting, of which I briefly observe in General, that they are sure to weaken or discompose when they are imployed, but do not certainly cure afterwards.[4]

Here Boyle was attacking Galen's general premise that evacuation was necessary to rid the body of a plethora of a specific humor and reestablish the humoral balance that was equated with the state of health. Boyle did not completely reject the notion that evacuative procedures could be appropriate; after all, this would be a way for the body to rid itself of the morbific matter that he felt was present in disease. But he insisted that a more feasible method of cure would be to administer a specific drug that acted locally to remove or neutralize the disease cause without putting the body as a whole in jeopardy.[5] He maintained, of course, that the development of such specialized cures required an experimental method based on chemical analysis.

Boyle's arguments clearly derived from the notion of equating disease with the alteration of texture, which he defined in both chemical and mechanical terms. Criticizing the overreliance on traditional evacuative procedures—phlebotomy, administration of cathartic or emetic drugs, and so on—Boyle warned that even a gentle evacuation may alter the ("chemical") constitution of the body. A "humour that would be morbific" but was previously "fettered" by the humor that now has been evacuated will now become "active and predominant and . . . able to do more harm than it could do before." Boyle further questioned the safety of the traditional method on mechanical grounds, noting that a purgative may do "mischief by agitating Noxious Humours that it does not evacuate" or "[awakening] some sleeping Ferment or some Peccant Humour, that lay quiet before, and by unseasonable or immoderate agitation, heightens it so as to become the Cause of a Disease."[6]

Although Boyle's own view of how nature operates led him to reject much of the traditional *methodus medendi,* he did not take the position that all principles underlying the existing method were false, nor that medicine should proceed without a method, as the empiric would have it.

> It was not my design . . . to subvert those principles of the *methodus medendi* from which no sober physicians themselves recede, and in which they unanimously acquiesce; and that I much less intend to countenance those venturous empiricks, who, without any competent knowledge of anatomy, botanicks, and the history of diseases, think receipts or processes alone can enable them to cure the sicknesses they know not, and who would persuade men to lay by, as needless, a profession, of whose usefulness to mankind, we may elsewhere have occasion to discourse.[7]

Rather, he maintained that the existing method of professional physicians was inadequate.

> It is not, that I am either an enemy to method in physick, or an undervaluer of it; but I fear the generality of physicians . . . have as yet but an imperfect method, and have by the narrow principles they were taught in the schools, been persuaded to change their method rather to the barren principles of the Peripatetick school, than to the full amplitude of nature. . . .

Boyle's Medical Thought in Context

> And indeed, it is scarce to be expected, that till men have a better knowledge of the principles of natural philosophy, without which it is hard to arrive at a more comprehensive theory of the various possible causes or diseases, and of the contrivance and uses of the parts of the body, the method which supposes this knowledge should be other than in many things defective, and in some erroneous.[8]

Although Boyle was convinced that the physician, like other investigators, would benefit from conceptualizing natural phenomena in terms of the mechanical motion of corpuscles rather than in terms of Aristotelian or Galenic "innate strivings" or "faculties," he rejected the idea of substituting an alternative medical method based on strict mechanical interpretations. He recognized that the specific needs of medical research required the formulation of lower-level hypotheses that could not necessarily be reduced to "mechanical" terms. In his *Certain Physiological Essays* Boyle specifically attacks those who would reject out of hand more qualitative hypotheses, not only to justify his own use of them but to legitimatize the work of "many learned men, *especially physicians,* whose useful writings [are] being undervalued, and are in danger to be despised, by an opinion taken up from the mis-understood doctrine of some eminent Atomists, as if no speculations in natural philosophy could be rational, wherein any other causes of things are assigned than atoms and their properties."[9]

Although lower-level hypotheses might be useful in all areas of scientific investigation, Boyle thought medicine was an area where such hypotheses could be particularly fruitful. For example, he maintained that a physician who investigated the particular qualities of a drug (particularly via chemical analysis) and then used that drug successfully in the treatment of disease possessed valid knowledge, even if he was unable to provide a meaningful explanation of the cause of the drug's efficacy in strict mechanistic terms. Most accepted medical practice, he noted, relied on hypotheses of this lower-level type.

> And as for the reasons of things assigned by physicians, they must be by most of them despised, unless we will allow of such explications, as deduce not things from atoms or their affections, but only either from secondary qualities, or from the more particular properties of mixt bodies. . . . And indeed, there are oftentimes so many subordinate causes between particular effects and the most general causes of things, that there is left a large field, wherein to exercise men's industry and reason, if they will but solidly enough deduce the properties of things from more general and familiar qualities, and also intermediate causes (if I may so call them) from one another.[10]

"Divulging of Useful Truths in Physick"

It was not requisite that discoveries by physicians or any other individual engaged in medical inquiry be accepted as valid only if they could be deduced from the most basic principles. Engaging in such lower-level inquiry not only had the advantage of expediency; it also allowed the investigator to "paint with more colors," to concentrate on a whole host of secondary qualities that a more rigorous inquiry into basic mechanics would require him, at least temporarily, to disregard.

Boyle's extensive writings on the subject of effluvia should be seen as his own articulation of a lower-level hypothesis, one with special relevance to medicine, especially in the areas of disease causation and drug action. He described effluvia chemically and qualitatively, and he derived causal hypotheses about specific effluvial activity from a variety of qualitative observations of their supposed effects. Boyle stated in his *Essays of the Strange Subtilty, great Efficacy, determinate Nature of Effluviums* that he hoped to show that this way of conceptualizing was compatible with his corpuscular hypothesis.[11] However, as a lower-level hypothesis, the concept of effluvial action included some assumptions that were not directly deducible from the first principles set forth in the corpuscular hypothesis. Examples of these are his postulations that all bodies contain pores and that all bodies emit effluvia.

Boyle's hypotheses about effluvia represent an effort on his part to bring *qualitative* considerations into an essentially mechanistic medical perspective. The corpuscular hypothesis itself might not provide the physician with a specific approach that could directly enhance his understanding and treatment of disease, but the formulation of effluvial penetration did establish a rationale for specific chemical investigation, which could prove more immediately profitable for medical practice. Since Boyle maintained that effluvial particles were chemically identical to the gross bodies from which they emanated, effluvia could be qualitatively differentiated. Even if their activities could not be observed directly, they could be described in terms of what was known about the chemistry of the gross substances from which they came. Since effluvia were aggregates of corpuscles, at the most basic level their actions were amenable to strict mechanical explanation. But chemistry, not mathematics, provided the greatest practical insight into their operations. (This commitment to practical science is the key to understanding why Boyle, unlike many other mechanists of his age, had little interest in promoting mathematical precision and preferred a more qualitative methodology.)

In positing effluvia as a lower-level hypothesis, Boyle was able to discuss qualitative submacroscopic interactions of matter while still maintaining the integrity of his mechanistic world-view. By forwarding essentially two different levels of explanation, Boyle was able to set himself apart from the tradition of Aristotelian minimists such as Daniel Sennert (1572–1637) and his nearer contemporary and associate Kenelm Digby, who, faced with the same problem as Boyle of making their theories of matter conducive to chemical explanations, had resorted to the postulate that the ultimate building blocks of matter, which they called minima, were themselves substantively and qualitatively different.[12] Although Boyle initially had envisioned minima much as Digby did, in his mature corpuscular philosophy he used the term "minima" to refer to the most basic class of corpuscles, which could not themselves be distinguished as chemically distinct. Only second-order corpuscles could be qualitatively differentiated.[13] Boyle's concept of effluvia is a good example of how Boyle, instead of rejecting explanations in terms of secondary qualities in favor of those based strictly on homogeneous matter in motion, accepted both types of explanations, simply by establishing as valid two separate levels of hypotheses.

Thus, used in a medical context, lower-level hypotheses would provide insights into effective treatments and afford plausible rationales for practical decision making. Medicine thereby would be based on probabilistic knowledge tied to experimental analysis. Rather than remaining a set of rigid principles, the *methodus medendi* would become a amalgam of hypotheses that would be improved over time. Such a flexible method would avoid the defects Boss described for the traditional one based on Galen, which could not itself change without compromising its utility. On the contrary, Boyle's view was that medical practice (and practical science) would be best served if new knowledge could be incorporated continuously. For Boyle, the goal was to augment and improve the existing *methodus medendi.*

Since such knowledge generation required the coordinated efforts of many investigators—to design experiments, validate findings, and agree upon acceptable interpretations of results—it was fitting that physicians allow themselves to engage in collaboration with the larger community of "natural philosophers" and not isolate their researches.[14] Boyle hoped in this way not only to reform medicine and improve the *methodus medendi* but to bring medicine into the larger domain of general scientific inquiry.

Contemporary Criticisms of Boyle's Approach

Despite Boyle's attempts to present his arguments in conciliatory fashion, he was not exempt from criticism. Contemporaries attacked his approach on professional, procedural, and philosophical grounds. For the educated physician, the prospect of coordinating research with those lacking formal medical training was viewed as threatening the very foundation of his professionalism. As Harold Cook has noted, some members of the Royal College of Physicians feared that if the virtuosi became deeply involved in medical investigations, as Boyle advocated, "the university-inculcated discipline of physic might become a merely curative art based upon empirically discovered therapies" and that such a transformation might "break down the division between the learned physicians and their unlearned rivals."[15]

Broadening the base of medical investigation to encompass findings in other areas of natural philosophy was itself seen as needlessly ambitious—and intrusive. Boyle and Henry Oldenburg deliberately had encouraged the Royal Society to take up such wide-scope investigations of relevance to medicine. In fact, according to Roy Porter, "general queries . . . aimed to stir up medical inquiry" were inserted in the *Philosophical Transactions* by Oldenburg with Boyle's assistance. Such queries, which indeed did prompt responses, touched upon areas of current medical controversy, such as the efficacy of mineral waters, or suggested topics for general "histories" of countries, which would shed light on possible relationships between climate and disease.[16] Yet overt efforts to encourage the general membership of the Royal Society to help broaden the scope of medical inquiry were ridiculed. An especially strong opponent of such wide-scope investigations was Baldwin Hamey, a member of the Royal College of Physicians. Hamey, as his biographer wrote, disapproved of a "Rival Society treading close upon the heels of the Aesculapians, whose vortex would be so great as to comprehend everything."[17] The implication was that it was preferable for the physician to retain control over a specialized area of knowledge gathering than to become inundated with (and intellectually paralyzed by) a tidal wave of unrelated facts on many subjects, only some of which would turn out to be truly relevant to either medical theory or medical practice.

Boyle, of course, continued to insist that a broadened perspective would benefit physicians in many ways. He argued that a greater familiarity with nature's operations would make the physician better aware of factors in the external environment that might affect disease, give him greater insights into substances that could be used as drugs, and provide intellectual fodder for developing novel hypotheses regarding physiological functioning. Boyle's *Usefulness of Experimental Natural Philosophy* stands as his testament to the many and varied ways medicine could be improved by wider-scope investigations. He no doubt believed that by enhancing his knowledge of nature, the physician would enhance his professional stature as well.

Boyle was, however, by no means ignorant of the fact that some physicians feared that their separate status as professionals would be compromised by the dabbling of virtuosi into medical matters. Boyle needed to allay such fears and yet still argue that natural philosophers had valuable contributions to make to medicine. He accomplished this in his published works by deliberately expressing his ideas on medicine with extreme caution and subtlety. He repeatedly reminded his readers that he was, after all, a layman, yet one who was anxious to make suggestions in the hope that professional physicians, who were more "knowledgeable" about medical matters, might find them useful and be willing to expand upon them on their own.[18]

By expressing himself in this deliberately humble and nondogmatic manner, Boyle hoped to attract a wide audience for his views. This style of presentation was also consistent with his opinion that knowledge should be presented as probabilistic, not certain. By insisting that knowledge generation was a long-term process, Boyle hoped to assuage any fears that medical reform would be sudden or impulsive or pose a threat to the existing social order. However, he ran the risk that his views would appear too tentative, and his method too long-term, at a time when the educated, licensed medical practitioners were desperate to distinguish themselves from the competition by finding a solid theoretical base for their practices in order to impress their patient clients and establish their professional credibility.

In addition to the concerns raised by physicians about the implications of Boyle's research agenda for their professional well-being, there were other very real concerns about the philosophical underpinnings of his approach. One particularly vocal opponent was Thomas Hobbes, who questioned Boyle's views on grounds that his experimental approach was logically faulty. The crux of Hobbes's opposition is based on what Maurice Mandelbaum has termed the "problem of transdiction," that is, "the question of how observed data can serve as the grounds for inferences to objects or events which not only have not yet been observed, but which cannot in principle be observed."[19] As Steven Shapin and Simon Schaffer have pointed out, Hobbes was not opposed to experiment "merely as a useful adjunct to the pursuit of natural philosophy"; rather, he was unwilling to accept the idea that any viable philosophy of nature must be grounded in experiment. Hobbes initially was prompted to criticize Boyle after the publication of Boyle's *New Experiments, Physico-Mechanical, Touching the Spring of the Air* in 1660. In this work Boyle's full-fledged experimental program for natural philosophy was articulated for the first time. Hobbes responded to Boyle in print with a treatise entitled *Dialogus physicus de natura aeris* in 1661.[20]

Shapin and Schaffer have provided a detailed account of Hobbes's criticisms of Boyle's experimental program, which will not be repeated here. Hobbes' arguments deal with Boyle's overall investigative approach and do not touch specifically upon his medical views. However, since Boyle's ideas on improving medical knowledge are part of his larger methodology, it is relevant to review Hobbes' criticisms briefly. Hobbes took issue both with the way experiments were performed and validated and with the propriety of using those results to make philosophical statements about the world. As to the conducting of experiments, Hobbes argued, among other things, that despite the rhetoric of obtaining *public* consensus on experimental findings, in reality those witnessing experiments constituted a private, self-selected group of associates; therefore, any consensus attained thereby should only be considered partial and limited.

Hobbes disagreed that universals proceeded from facts, and therefore he insisted that no experimental program could never reveal the first principles underlying nature. He also maintained that the experimental program of Boyle short-circuited the proper method of philosophical inquiry, which could proceed only insofar as one could establish consensus on metaphysical language. Further, Hobbes felt that it was "unphilosophical" to try to establish a procedural boundary between observing facts and identifying basic causes. While Boyle maintained that hypotheses derived from experiments should be considered conjectural only, "in Hobbes view, in order to be counted as philosophy an intellectual practice could not affect nescience concerning the causes of things."[21]

Boyle, of course, rejected Hobbes criticisms. His *Examen of Hobbes's Dialogus* (1662) was but the first of Boyle's responses to Hobbes. Despite his aversion to confrontation, Boyle was willing to respond to Hobbes's criticism because he feared that Hobbes's fame and self-assured writing style might prejudice people against experimental philosophy. Boyle not only aimed to counter Hobbes's criticisms; he used the opportunity of publishing a response to "give a concrete demonstration of how disputes ought to be managed and brought to a conclusion."[22]

Boyle defended the value and integrity of the experimental program, accusing Hobbes of undeservedly undermining the Royal Society and also, by inference, impugning the moral character of the gentlemen who witnessed experiments and provided testimony concerning the validity of experimental findings. Boyle maintained that since Hobbes had not performed experiments himself, he could not fully understand the process of knowledge gathering that Boyle approved. He pointed out the dogmatic aspect of Hobbes's views, noting the inappropriateness of such a position for scientific dialogue. He also argued against Hobbes on theological grounds, challenging his views as diminishing God's role by rendering God incapable of giving men assurance of his existence and of his providence. He pointed out the defects in Hobbes's alternative interpretations of some of Boyle's specific views of nature, for example, regarding the creation of a vacuum or an explanation of the air's "elasticity." In short, Boyle criticized Hobbes for ignorance of the rules of ongoing scientific inquiry and for being himself logically inconsistent. Clearly, Boyle was anxious to counter Hobbes's attack on the fundamental basis of his experimental methodology.

In addition to the critical views expressed by Hobbes, there was another challenge to Boyle's methodology, one with direct implications for medicine. This was the argument that broadly focused research and attempts to develop tentative hypotheses regarding the most basic operations of nature simply could not provide adequate guidance to the physician for his day-to-day practice. Those holding this position declared their preference for a method more confined to direct clinical observation and classification. The philosophical discussions forwarded in support of this viewpoint focused both on the "proper" goal of medicine and on the limits of human knowledge.

Boyle's contemporary Thomas Sydenham was among those arguing for a narrower focus of investigation. Although Sydenham rejected Boyle's idea that the goals of medicine would be served by greatly expanding the physician's perspective, he and Boyle actually agreed on many other things relating to medicine. The two men were good friends. Sydenham was at Oxford when Boyle was performing experiments there in the mid-1650s. In the late 1660s Sydenham lived next-door to Boyle's sister Katherine, Lady Ranelagh, in London. Boyle and Sydenham had long been in contact with each other by this time; Boyle had even accompanied Sydenham on visits to patients. Sydenham shared with Boyle a belief in the value of an empirical approach, an interest in a therapeutics-based medicine (based on drug simples), and especially the idea that airborne morbific particles operating at the corpuscular level could cause a variety of diseases.[23] Andrew Cunningham has suggested that Boyle may have instigated Sydenham's initial investigation of epidemic fever and has noted that Sydenham's approach reflects much of Boyle's influence.[24] Nonetheless, the two men came to differ on some fundamental points.

Sydenham completely rejected both the possibility of comprehending the underlying operations of nature and the necessity of obtaining such knowledge. He believed that one's search for the hidden causes of nature led only to phantasmal speculations and diverted one's attention from the "proper" task of obtaining practical information through gross observations. Ultimate causes in nature, according to Sydenham, were comprehensible only to God himself; for a human being to presume to understand them was vanity. Thus the investigator was to adopt a posture of passive dependence upon God, admitting that the human capacity to know nature was very limited, so limited, in fact, that the *only* type of information individuals could rely on was that discernible by the senses God saw fit to give them. Sydenham believed that physicians should confine their observations to the "outer husk of things," since God had designed their senses only to perceive that much. Because of this view, Sydenham rejected the use of vision-enhancing tools such as the microscope in scientific investigation, insisting that the view of the world obtained thereby was merely artificial and provided no practical information, only more fodder for speculation.

Sydenham was convinced that medical progress could be achieved only through the accumulation of factual data directly appropriate to the physician's craft. Since the heart of that craft was the careful observation of the patient and determination of appropriate remedies, he emphasized the importance of amassing clinical observations. From such observations, one could draw correlations and derive accurate pictures of the symptoms and course of specific diseases and of the cures empirically found to be most effective for each. Sydenham held that even if one could discern the first principles of nature, this knowledge would provide no practical information. On similar grounds, he maintained that only a general knowledge of anatomy was necessary for the physician. Detailed anatomical investigation, however interesting, rendered nothing practical to medicine, since insights into function could never be gained by investigating structure. Sydenham's essentially antireductionist attitude led him to insist that the proper task for the physician was to compile histories of disease based solely upon repeated clinical observations.

While Boyle hoped that systematic investigation and data collection would yield insights into the basic operations of nature, Sydenham limited himself to the realm of the observable. The boundary between experiment and theory, which Boyle had recognized but hoped to bridge with his own carefully constructed program of hypothesis formulation and verification, became for Sydenham an insurmountable barrier between what man could know and what God alone could know. Sydenham's hypotheses were judged in terms of their consistency with each other, not in terms of their compatibility with any higher-order generalized hypothesis.

Sydenham's goal was to utilize extensive clinical observations to discover definitive symptomatic patterns for identifying diseases; he wanted to categorize disease species. Once this classification was accomplished, the physician would have an immediately practical means by which to determine how to diagnose and treat individual patients. As Sydenham's close friend John Locke noted in a letter to Dr. Thomas Molyneux, the "hypotheses" derived from Sydenham's disease histories "served as an art of memory" for the physician.[25]

Sydenham's focus and intent were quite different from those of Boyle's open-ended inquiry. While Sydenham's method emphasized categorization and had little heuristic emphasis, Boyle insisted that

> till men have a better knowledge of the principles of natural philosophy, without which it is hard to arrive at a more comprehensive theory of the various possible causes of diseases, and of the contrivance and uses of the parts of the body, the method which supposes this knowledge should be other than in many things defective, and in some erroneous.[26]

Sydenham maintained, however, that

> wise and learned . . . as [the doctor] may be, he will do no real good in medicine, who, instead of investigating the . . . methods whereby Nature evolves disease, instead of studying their history, and instead of putting forth his whole strength to the adaptation of remedies, wearies his brain with curious and irrelevant speculations; speculations which, for the proper undertaking of medicine, the saving of men from death are not one iota of value.[27]

It is particularly interesting that Boyle and Sydenham both argued their cases from the standpoint of theology. For Boyle, God intended for people to inquire into his design as an act of veneration. Individuals, secure in their faith that a design exists and that God wishes them to perceive it, establish hypotheses by which they can, in their limited way, perceive nature as a holistic, interrelated creation. In this effort they are free to use not only the "light of reason" provided them by God but any other tools God has made available to them or allowed them to invent by their own hands. By extending their sense perception in these ways, people can obtain a fuller picture of the natural order that underlies specific events. Such knowledge leads to better hypotheses concerning particular operations of nature, which lead to practical improvements.

In Sydenham's interpretation, God encourages one less to contemplate his design than to submit oneself to it. Human beings must know their place and must not aspire to knowledge beyond their purview. To carry out God's design, they must dedicate themselves to good works, using their limited capabilities as best they can to achieve tangible results. For physicians, this meant that they should, by their own powers of observation, classify their clinical findings and thereby devise a modus operandi that had immediate applicability for the performance of their craft. This classification need not be "true" in a universal sense, yet its artificiality should not prevent it from being a useful organizational device for determining therapy. Like the craftsman, one need not know the true nature of the materials one worked on to create something with them.

Boyle, however, equated classification with system building and foresaw dangers of dogmatizing. The rigid structuring of nature that classification fostered might well organize knowledge but might also result in impeding it by limiting one's vision, particularly with regard to new information. Like Galen, Sydenham felt that what was knowable in medicine was already known or at hand, just waiting to be codified. Boyle's much broader view of medical knowledge, which involved an understanding of the overall operations of nature, necessitated that one not systematize too soon, lest one be deluded by partial comprehension into drawing false conclusions.

Boyle was especially concerned "to beget a good understanding betwixt the chymists and the mechanical philosophers," a view Sydenham did not share. Sydenham's approach, after all, was best engaged in by those specifically trained in medicine.[28] Boyle held great hope that a chemical understanding of the body would be of tremendous value to the physician. Chemical analysis employed to ascertain the basic properties of substances, he hoped, would further the general understanding of the body both in sickness and in health and would underscore the fact that material, not occult, causes were at work. Through observation and experiment, one could build up a body of knowledge that could augment and ultimately reform medicine. Sydenham was not as optimistic concerning the practical benefits of such a chemical perspective. He recognized that much chemical work was highly speculative and therefore would turn the physician's attention away from the direct observation of the patient.

John Locke, also a physician, forwarded arguments similar to those of Sydenham. However, Locke was more interested in exploring the limits of knowledge than in devising a specific agenda for medical inquiry. Like Sydenham, Locke chose to focus on the realm of the directly observable. He felt that the task of the natural philosopher was to make a more thorough investigation of what one can know through one's senses and to organize that information for practical purposes. Although Locke did not deny the existence of a realm of reality beyond the senses, he maintained that that realm was so uncertain and our knowledge was so limited that it was best to concentrate on the realm of the more knowable and not to try to bridge the gap between the observed world and the more basic realm of ultimate reality, even by the modest means of devising "plausible" hypotheses.

Patrick Romanell, in his analysis of the relationship of Locke's medical views to his overall philosophy, suggests that ironically it was Locke's acceptance of Boyle's corpuscular hypothesis, with its persuasive argument that the basic operations of nature take place at a subvisible level, that led to Locke's conviction that nature was inscrutable. As Romanell remarks, citing Locke's *Essay Concerning Human Understanding:* "[Locke] is so *certain* about the 'insensible' constituents of nature that he is forced to become *uncertain* about our knowledge of them. To know them we would need . . . to be blessed or cursed with 'microscopical eyes.'"[29]

Locke, like Sydenham, maintained that the only proper goal of medical inquiry was the practical one of determining cures; the test of any hypotheses generated in medicine could only be whether or not it was valid for therapy. Locke, labeled by Romanell a "medical pragmatist," draws a sharp distinction between the "practicing physician" and the "medical scientist." The patient seeks out a "doctor," not a "biologist," when treatment is needed. Where Boyle wished to integrate medicine into science, Locke seeks to keep them separate. He believed that the physician has a defined, practical mission from which he should not be deterred by conjecturing upon possible underlying mechanisms of nature. Such speculation leads to bias, not insight. Locke believed that the primary deficiency of traditional medicine was its lapse into such flights of imaginative "fancies." Even if such speculations were held, as Boyle insisted, to be probable only, and not certain, they still represented for Locke an unprofitable detour that hurt more than it helped the progress of medicine, since it diverted the physician from his primary professional responsibilities.

Because Locke both limited medicine's proper sphere of inquiry and maintained an agnostic position concerning the possibility of developing a rational metaphysics, his views on the conduct of scientific investigation, even within the realm of the observable, differed from Boyle's. For example, again like Sydenham, he denied that anatomy was of much use to the practice of medicine. In a manuscript fragment "Anatomia," written in 1668, Locke, following Sydenham, described the inappropriateness of anatomical investigation to medicine.

> The laborious anatomist I will not deny knows more, but not more to the purpose [of knowing diseases and their cure], for if he cannot come to dis-

cover these little differences which preserve health or make a disease, if he cannot possibly see how nature prepares those juices which serve in their fitt places and proportions for the use and preservation of the body he may perhaps be the better anatomist by multiplying dissections, but not a better physician.

Boyle had urged the study of anatomy because it would serve as a visual tool, providing insights into the design of the body and spurring the formulation of broader and more ingenious hypotheses about nature's operations. Locke, however, specifically rejected this idea that anatomical visualization advantages medicine: "For could the intent looking upon any part teach us to cure its diseases then ladys would have more reason to go to the painter than physician for the removal of freckles and scabs, sore eyes, and sallow cheeks from their faces." What Locke saw as a useful tool for the practicing physician was not an improved vision of the body but improved *memory.* He maintained that the observation of diseases would allow the physician to "'frame' some tentative 'ideas' about their 'causes or their ways of operation,' in other words, some hypothesis that, 'though not perhaps true in its self yet will be a great help to his memory and a guid to his practise.'"[30]

Locke's emphasis on the mneumonic value of hypotheses is reiterated in a letter to Dr. Thomas Molyneux of 20 January 1692/93, where he wrote: "Upon such grounds as are the establish'd history of diseases hypotheses might with less danger be erected, which I think are so far useful, as they serve as an *art of memory* to direct the physician in particular cases, but not to be rely'd on as foundations of reasoning, or verities to be contended for."[31]

Locke's position that the knowledge-gathering process is limited constitutes a fundamental difference between his "use" of lower-level hypotheses and Boyle's. While Boyle agreed with Locke that lower-level hypotheses have value in producing guidelines immediately useful to medical practice, he also saw such hypotheses as capable of refinement, as eventually providing suggestions about the underlying workings of nature. For Locke, however, lower-level hypotheses never became more than a practical set of statements, hence his emphasis on their value to the memory rather than to their ultimate potential for yielding general insights into nature.

Even while Locke, like Sydenham, insisted that knowledge could be augmented solely by investigation of the "outer husks of things," he was much more pessimistic about the outcome. Unlike Sydenham, Locke did not hold that the results of our correlation of information would yield real categories, such as disease species. Locke realized the artificiality of classification in a way Sydenham did not. He simply accepted the notion that "plausible" categorization (of observed phenomena) could be a useful means of organizing information that could aid therapeutic decision making.

The primary distinction, then, between Locke's views and those of Boyle has to do with expectations. Locke the pragmatist viewed knowledge as limited and the goal of medicine as circumscribed. Boyle maintained an eclectic, inclusivist position, aiming to bring medicine within the larger sphere of science. "Health" for Locke meant simply the absence of disease in an individual. Boyle also saw health as the primary goal of medicine, but for him it had a host of metaphysical implications regarding harmony in nature's operations, the improvement of the human condition, the fulfillment of God's intentions for humanity, and even the maintenance of social order. It was these broader ramifications that not only prompted Boyle's intense interest in medicine but also legitimized his efforts to subsume medicine within the larger framework of natural philosophy. Although his critics might argue against the practicality of his approach or the logic of his method, Boyle maintained that his suggestions for the improvement of medicine would at the very least spur new and varied investigative efforts.

Recommendations for Research

Boyle believed that physicians, like natural philosophers, would benefit from organizing their information and developing a "history" of their subject—the human body. Toward this end, he developed, in a fragment contained in one of his notebooks, a set of titles appropriate to such a history. These titles, which really name suggested areas for research, reveal clearly that he viewed the study of the human body in much the same terms as he viewed the study of other complex phenomena in nature: a full examination required both a chemical and a mechanical accounting of the subject under consideration.

> Among the things by me suggested or recommended to Trallianus were these and such like:
>
> • The History of the Liquors of the Body, as blood, chyle, serum, lympha, gaul, *succus pancreaticus,* etc.
>
> • The Chymico-mechanical History of ye Firm or Stable (or consistent) parts of the Body: as Bones, Flesh, Tendons, Ligaments, Parenchymatous parts (as ye Liver, Splene, Kidneys etc). All which parts are here to be con-

sider'd as to their bulke, weight, situation, etc. and as to the different substances they yield upon Chymical Analyses of them: as also to their figurations and proportions of Bulk and weight to one another, among those that are coherent, as are the distinct humours and coals of the Eye.

- The History of the Invisible Fluids of the Body such as the Spirits, Animal and Vital, the Ferments, either properly so called, or Analogous.
- The Imitation (by way of Production) of morbific matters.
- The Artificial production of Diseases in the Bodys of Animals.
- The History of the secretions of a human Body; as Urine, the *Excrementa alvi,* sweat, spittle, snott. To which head may be reduc'd what is discharged by insensible transpiration.
- The History of digestion which is a part [of] Alimentation, showing the series of changes, or ye alterations that the Aliment undergoes from the time 'tis taken in at the mouth, til it be assimilated to the several parts of the Body.
- The chymico-mechanical Examen, or History of several aliments, whether Solid or Liquid.
- The Historical Analysis of Egges.[32]

Here, as he had done frequently on other scientific topics, Boyle presented a host of suggestions dealing with how medical research should be conducted and what avenues might be most promising in achieving greater understanding of disease and cure. His aim was to provide investigators with a set of questions, not answers.

Boyle's suggestions for various investigations into the human body and the intriguing hypotheses his own personal research generated did elicit interest among those who came after him. Even those who criticized his overall methodology were willing to admit that Boyle had provided physicians with some useful notions.

Boyle's Medical Thought in Context

CHAPTER SEVEN

Boyle's Legacy

Boyle's "Medical" Reputation

It is difficult to assess how much Boyle's views specifically influenced later medical writers, since his work often closely mirrors that of others in the scientific community of his own day. In addition, he was extremely solicitous not to appear confrontational toward the professional medical community; as a result, he conveyed his medical thoughts with careful subtlety, usually adding that he would not presume to dictate to physicians, that he only wished to forward interesting suggestions and speculations. This deliberately tentative style was probably due more to Boyle's anxiety not to incur the wrath of professional physicians than to any real feelings of inadequacy.

Moreover, as Harold Cook has explained, intellectuals of the mid-seventeenth century became increasingly cautious in their quarrels with each other, lest the general public lose respect for learning altogether.[1] It was hard enough to maintain traditional ideas of professional stature and social standing in this changeable age. Boyle, of course, as a member of the upper class, had a vested interest in seeing the existing social order maintained. He was also anxious to avoid becoming associated with those critics—mostly iatrochemists—then attacking both medicine's theoretical foundations and its institutional makeup, who were urging an immediate and total restructuring of the discipline.

The Royal College of Physicians in London was at its weakest between 1660 and 1672. It was unable to exhibit any strong regulatory control and was itself divided by internal dissension among its members.[2] These were, of course, the years when the new Royal Society of London was most active and when Boyle was writing and doing research on topics related to medicine. His *Usefulness of Experimental Natural Philosophy* was published in 1663, with a second edition a year later. The work was evidently quite popular. He also was becoming identified with the work being done on respiration at Oxford. His *New Experiments, Physico-Mechanical, Touching the Spring of the Air* first appeared in 1660. Therefore, people were aware of his medical interests and willing to listen to what he had to say.

It was important to Boyle to maintain a conciliatory position. Cook points out that in the preface to *Usefulness of Experimental Natural Philosophy* Boyle says he was "'restrained by some justifiable Considerations' from setting down all the chemical experiments of use to physicians, 'especially 'till I see what Entertainment, the things I now venture abroad, will meet with there.'"[3] Boyle needed to make it especially clear that his views, especially those involving greater participation of chemists in medical inquiry, should not be construed as support for Paracelsian or Helmontian medicine, with its emphasis on occult qualities and directive forces in nature, or for pure trial-and-error empiricism. Not only did he believe that these approaches were faulty and limited but he knew that the more conservative professional physicians strongly resisted such approaches, especially since they were being advocated by those most outspoken about the need for immediate and total medical reform. Boyle sought accommodation, not revolution. As an advocate of social order, he never questioned the institutional basis of medical professionalism. He simply wished to persuade formally educated physicians to accept a broader perspective and to be more open to new ideas. His hope was for gradual change through reasoned discussion.

Because of Boyle's conciliatory demeanor and growing reputation as a capable scientist, he was read by a wide audience and respected by the intellectual community. By the end of the 1660s he had become quite famous. It is noteworthy that at the time Boyle was gaining this fame, he was deeply involved in work relevant to medicine. In addition to publishing works emphasizing the utility of the experimental approach to medicine and conducting innovative experiments on respiration using the air pump, he was actively engaged in pharmacological work and investigations into the chemical aspects of digestion.[4] By the end of the 1660s he had also become involved in injection and transfusion experiments. Other medical authors honored Boyle by dedicating their own writings to him. Some of these works were major contributions to medicine, such as the *Diatribae Thomae Willisii . . . de Febribus Vindicatio* (1666), by his Oxford colleague Richard Lower, and Walter Needham's *Disquisitio anatomica formato foetu* (1667).

Boyle's advice on medical matters was sought frequently, even by practicing physicians. In the plague year of 1665, Hugh Chamberlen, of the famous Chamberlen family of physicians, sent Boyle a copy of his "Essay of the Plague" and asked whether he had any better suggestions on how to rid London of the epidemic.[5] Maddison notes that Boyle seems to have been especially highly regarded (and frequently consulted) for his knowledge of the eye. It is true that Boyle added an appendix entitled "Some Uncommon Observations about Vitiated Sight" to his 1688 treatise *A Disquisition about the final Causes of Natural Things* in order to "gratify a philosophical physician."[6] Samuel Pepys regarded him as having expertise in eye disorders, and according to Maddison, "even Dr. Daubeney Turberville, when in doubt, would send a patient to him for examination."[7]

Given Boyle's increasing recognition for his knowledge of medical matters by the mid-1660s, it is not surprising that he was awarded an honorary medical degree from Oxford in 1665. The date itself is significant, for it was only a year after the successful publication of the second edition of *Usefulness of Experimental Natural Philosophy,* the work that provides his most direct statements on improvement of the medical art.

Although not all Boyle's associates accepted his experimental philosophy *in toto,* a number of them did become interested in making investigations along some of the lines he had advocated. An overview of late-seventeenth- and early eighteenth-century medicine reveals that specific ideas and avenues of research that Boyle suggested in his writings extended well beyond his time. This was partly due to parallel development, of course, since the direction of Boyle's work was shaped by the medical problems current in his day and by the interests of his medical colleagues. However, Boyle's work is credited specifically by several of these later investigators, indicating that at least some researchers, including physicians, of the generation after Boyle were receptive to his particular formulations or inspired by his recommendations for further inquiry.

Expanding Foundations of Medical Investigation: The Institutional Perspective

During Boyle's lifetime, his desire to see physicians and nonmedically trained virtuosi collaborate more closely was at least to some degree fulfilled, although not necessarily in the way he expected. Among the active membership of the Royal Society during its early years were a number of medical men. Michael Hunter has estimated that of the 479 fellows elected between 1660 and 1700, 16 percent were medical practitioners. This figure does not include those, like Christopher Wren, who were trained in medicine but whose careers followed a nonmedical path.[8]

Experiments relevant to medicine accounted for almost half of all experiments performed in the Royal Society's early decades.[9]

A number of the physicians who were members of the early Royal Society also held membership in the Royal College of Physicians. Such men included Walter Charleton, Christopher Merrett, Jonathan Goddard, William Petty, and William Croune, the first registrar of the Royal Society. A. R. Hall suggests that during these years about one-fifth of the members of the Royal College were also members of the Royal Society.[10] Upon the establishment of the Royal Society in 1660, there had been an expectation that close relations would develop between the Royal Society and the Royal College. This was not to be the case, due both to the Royal Society's desire to assert its scientific independence and to the troubles plaguing the Royal College regarding its power to regulate and the need to reach agreement concerning the degree to which the incorporation of new ideas into the discipline was justified. There was from the outset the fear that the Royal Society was encroaching too much upon the physicians' domain.

Some physicians chose to challenge this negative view and to insist that the ideas of the new science and the benefits of collaborative research with the Royal Society could advantage the profession. Christopher Merrett, who held membership in both the Royal Society and the Royal College, exemplifies this position. Although he was not very involved in the activities of the Royal Society during its first two years, he came to be a vocal advocate for an eclectic perspective in medicine and for joint research between physicians and virtuosi.[11] After the London fire of 1666, Merrett even proposed, unsuccessfully, that the Royal Society and the Royal College build a common meeting hall.

The Royal College's suspicions toward the Royal Society continued to grow, however. Works praising the experimental approach and the activities of the Royal Society, such as Thomas Sprat's *History of the Royal Society* (1667) and Joseph Glanvill's *Plus Ultra* (1668), increased, rather than defused, the fears of the Royal College. Merrett's own attempts to deflect the increasing criticism and direct the blame for professional encroachment toward the apothecaries were not widely successful.[12] The lines of conflict deepened when the acerbic Henry Stubbe was convinced to publish a reply to Sprat and Glanvill in 1670. Stubbe probably entered the fray at the urging of Baldwin Hamey, a "traditionalist" within the Royal College.[13]

With the publication of Stubbe's scathing works—"The Plus Ultra Reduced to a Non Plus" and "Legends no Histories: Or, A Specimen of

Some Animadversions Upon the History of the Royal Society"—the hope for reconciliation between the two organizations dimmed. A pamphlet war began, with the apothecaries also appearing in print to defend themselves against what they saw as unfair criticisms of their work by both the Royal College and the community of experimental scientists.

Under such conditions, opportunities for harmonious collaborations between medical professionals and gentlemen virtuosi became more and more limited. By the time the Royal College of Physicians regained its power during the reign of James II and once again exercised regulatory control over the professional physicians in London, the medical activities within the Royal Society had declined. Even by the late 1660s and early 1670s few physicians remained active in the Royal Society, and almost no demonstrations in physiology were performed in the 1670s.[14]

Cook suggests that this decline in medical-related activity was due to the withdrawal of physicians from the Royal Society and the society's subsequent inability to recruit new ones because academic physicians perceived the new science to be a professional threat.

> The problem was clear by 1668. The challenge of the empirical science promoted by members of the Royal Society and others could not be entirely co-opted by the learned physicians if they wished to stress a knowledge of the academic medical traditions as being important to physic. They could not control a scientific medicine; such a medical program allowed empirics to claim that experimentalism was better than the education of the learned physicians. . . . By the 1660s, it had become clear to some that the new science might undermine the status of learned men as often as it might better it.[15]

This is certainly not the vision Boyle had in mind. Although his program of research was not limited to any single group, he obviously hoped to engage the educated "elite" among physicians in continuing dialogue, for this would be the best way to legitimize reforms at the highest professional level. Any successful revamping of medicine would require the strong support of the Royal College.

Boyle was certainly aware of physicians' growing opposition toward the virtuosi. The period of strained relations with the Royal College of Physicians and the medical practitioners' declining participation in the Royal Society came in the late 1660s. Boyle had permanently relocated to London from Oxford in 1668. He may indeed have become even more cautious in statements in work published in this later stage of his life about how nonmedically trained investigators could augment medical knowledge.

A. R. Hall has indicated that there *is* a difference in the tone between Boyle's early and his later work. Hall asserts (too forcefully, however) that "in his earlier years . . . Boyle showed a rather nonchalant inclination to criticize unspecified physicians for excessive narrowness or caution." As evidence he cites Boyle's statement in part 2 of *Usefulness of Experimental Natural Philosophy* that the naturalist could help the physician by providing explanations of the operations of specific drugs that hitherto physicians had failed to use because their mode of operation was unknown.[16] Hall interprets this as assigning to the physician the role of pupil and the naturalist the role of teacher, but it is perhaps better to interpret Boyle's statement here and elsewhere in that work as one promoting free communication between equals. This view would be consistent with Boyle's youthful idealism and his strong association with Hartlib and the utopian vision of Hartlib's circle at the time he was drafting *Usefulness of Experimental Natural Philosophy.*

As Hall correctly points out, however, Boyle's statements in a much later treatise, *Of the Reconcileableness of Specific Medicines to the Corpuscular Philosophy* (1685), convey a much greater respect for the physician's professional expertise.[17] In the introduction to this work, Boyle acknowledges that he is treating his subject, the efficacy of specific drugs,

> less like a physician than a naturalist; for . . . the medicinal art, and this science [i.e., natural philosophy] will be conversant about the same subject, though in differing ways, and with differing scopes; for there are divers hurtful or advantageous accidents and changes of the human body, whereof the naturalist takes notice, but as they are phaenomena or changes produced by natural causes in the body of an animal, whilst the physician considers them as symptoms of diseases, or effects of medicine: the former directs his speculations to the discovery of truth, and the other his theory to the recovery of health.[18]

Here Boyle is careful to distinguish the practicing physician from the medical scientist. As noted in chapter 6, John Locke also argued that there was a fundamental difference between the two. But while in Locke's case the distinction was used to define limits of inquiry for each, Boyle is attempting to validate the physician's own unique perspective while still maintaining that the natural philosopher's contributions can be instructive. There is yet an opportunity for dialogue. Boyle has not strayed from his convictions that collaborative effort is justified; he is simply tempering his comments to avoid any inference that he is encroaching upon the physician's professional territory. Collaboration between equals will still be possible, but, he insists, the particular expertise of each will be respected. He may well have thought it necessary to stress this point because of the Royal College's animosity toward experimental science at the time.

The Changing Character of Medicine

Although united experimental efforts by virtuosi and physicians were never undertaken on the large scale Boyle had envisioned, medicine nonetheless underwent significant change in the decades following Boyle's death. Unlike the seventeenth century, which had seen such bitter professional rivalries, the eighteenth century was a period of codification of new medical ideas, proliferation of medical "systems," a shift to a secularized, rational perspective, and the adoption of a more managerial and interventionist approach to the treatment of disease. Although Boyle himself would have questioned the wisdom of the system building that was taking place, he doubtless would have approved the development of a more eclectic, nonconfrontational attitude on the part of physicians. He also would have agreed with the greater emphasis on social welfare and public health that marked Enlightenment medicine.

Many of the specific changes that characterized eighteenth century medicine were consistent with Boyle's vision for medical reform. Disease was now commonly interpreted as a natural condition. There was a continued interest in localized therapy and in the use of simples, rather than compound drugs. The physician was permitted greater latitude and was less tied to traditional authority than in the past.

On the theoretical side, there was considerable interest in the environment's effects on health. One might speak, in fact, of a "Hippocratic renaissance" from the time of Sydenham on into the eighteenth century. Interest in meteorology as well as miasmic "airs" from damps and mines and sanative "airs" compounded in mineral waters was keen in eighteenth-century medicine. Physicians were willing to view body processes in terms of dynamic interactions of corpuscles, and in accordance with Newtonian physics, they rapidly extended these views to include the operation of short-range forces.

Pneumatics, which had occupied so much of Boyle's time, became a strong focus of much eighteenth-century scientific thought, and one that had obvious implications for medicine. The hydraulic imagery used to conceptualize body functions continued to be used from Harvey's time to Boyle's to Newton's, becoming incorporated into the medical theories of the great synthesizer of medical thought, Hermann Boerhaave. The perception of disease as consisting in morbific particles insinuating themselves within the body and requiring mollification or removal also continued into the eighteenth century. There was also a continuation of the literature on the chemical composition of mineral waters, much of it focusing on the need for more systematic methods of analysis, something Boyle also had emphasized and responded to in his own work on that subject.

Expanding Foundations of Medical Investigation: Specific Areas of Research

A number of trained physicians came forth to take the lead in improving the medical art. Corpuscular views provided a fundamental philosophical base for the theoretical perspectives of many, and Boyle directly inspired some. References to Boyle in works of later medical writers reveal their familiarity with his ideas on broad research, the use of both chemical and mechanical interpretations in physiology, and the cultivation of harmonious relations among investigators.

Boyle's ideas relating health and disease to particulate interactions between the human body and its environment were articulated and extended in various ways. As already noted, Boyle's colleague Thomas Sydenham extended and elaborated ideas that related disease to meteorological conditions, utilizing notions of subterraneal effluvial activity and viewing disease in terms of morbific particles in ways very similar to those of Boyle.

Another interesting example of how theoretical ideas such as Boyle's were translated into medical philosophy in the late seventeenth and early eighteenth centuries is the work of Friedrich Hoffmann. Hoffmann, born at Halle in 1660, spent some time in close association with Boyle in England during the early 1680s. Hoffmann became professor of medicine at the newly established University of Halle and during his lifetime attempted to establish a new system of medicine that would provide a rationale for the physician's practical decision making.

Lester King has discussed the shortcomings of Hoffmann's too-facile reductionism and premature systematization;[19] it is noteworthy, however, that many ideas similar to Boyle's found their way into Hoffmann's work. Hoffmann begins his *Fundamenta Medicinae* (1695) with the following optimistic declaration:

> Without natural philosophy the whole science of healing is maimed and weak. . . . Mechanics alone, wedded to anatomy and chemistry, has so far led natural and medical science from a low position to an exalted one.

Whoever has been properly instructed in such science can, in a most successful fashion, ferret out the causes of hidden matters; resolve the doubts of physicians, their controversies and opinions; find powerful remedies even in incurable diseases.[20]

Maintaining an essentially mechanistic view, Hoffmann particularly emphasized motion as a ruling principle of the body. In his eight-volume major work on medicine, *Medicina rationalis systematica* (1729–39), he writes:

We learn by careful observation that motion is the cause of all bodily changes, that in motion also lies the basis of life and health; that the very causes of diseases act upon the solid and fluid parts of our body in no other way than through motion; nor do therapeutic agents exert their effect except by motion. Therefore, in explaining medical phenomena and therapeutic activity, we consider that special attention should be paid to motion, and to motility or the disposition of bodies [to movement], and their pathways.[21]

This is very close to Boyle's own vision of the body as an inertial system that underwent change due to changes in motion. Further, Hoffmann clearly interprets life and death as a continuum, as did Boyle, relating in a summary passage that "life and death are mechanically conditioned and depend only on mechanical and physical causes which act by necessary laws."[22] This passage also reveals Hoffmann's rejection of the directive power of the soul, which prompted his opposition to the work of his vitalist colleague at Halle, Peter Staehl. Like Boyle, Hoffmann viewed life processes as emerging from the God-created structure of the body itself. Since the human body obeyed natural laws, Hoffmann, like Boyle, saw no need to posit directive "faculties," "plastic powers," or "occult virtues" as the source of activity. Hoffmann countered Staehl's view that the soul was a necessary "external" source of motion by insisting that it was, in fact, unneeded, since the motion in the body was self-perpetuating (i.e., built into the design).[23] Hoffmann, again like Boyle, urged the study of anatomy as the best way of gaining insight into the dynamic configuration of the body.

Where Hoffmann parts company with Boyle is in suggesting that all motions within the body can be referred ultimately to the contraction and expansion of nervous and muscular fibers. This idea becomes translated into the practical dictum that the physician must focus specifically on restoring the free motion and circulation of the blood to achieve cures from disease.[24] Although Boyle might have agreed in principle with this view, he certainly would not have approved of associating the restoration of texture *exclusively* with improving blood circulation.

If corpuscular ideas such as Boyle's can be seen as finding expression in the work of later medical writers, so can his interest in reconciling warring parties and creating a peaceful climate for research. The work of Hermann Boerhaave, the most respected synthesizer of medical thought of the eighteenth century, exemplifies this viewpoint. Eighteenth-century physicians' tendency to develop comprehensive systems of medicine (often based on a few simple principles) usually reflects their desire for greater certainty in medicine than would have been possible had they followed Boyle's admonition to build up a large body of knowledge without drawing premature conclusions. Boerhaave's aim, however, was to reduce conflict and promote peace among physicians by devising and organizing a comprehensive (and eclectic) set of rationales for treatment. Cunningham suggests that at root, Boerhaave's efforts should be seen as an expression of a religious attitude he clearly shared with Boyle—irenicism. In fact, Boerhaave encouraged physicians to pursue their investigations in an open-minded manner and to avoid preconceptions, which lead to the perversion of truth.[25]

Boerhaave's own work emphasized—not without considerable value judgment—the similarity between the doctrines of Hippocrates and the early Greek physicians and those of such moderns as Harvey and Sydenham. An investigation of history would uncover the "core truths" of medicine that all good authorities held in common. Using this historical perspective, a "system" of medicine could be created that would embody basic principles on which all contemporary physicians could agree. Boerhaave's debt to Bacon, whom he cited as an exemplar of good scientific procedure, is obvious. Boerhaave also singled out Boyle's own work for praise. He noted Boyle's careful attention to experiment and the caution with which Boyle forwarded his conclusions, saying: "No body ever made more experiments, or with more care and caution, than he. . . . He is ever exceedingly wary and reserved in drawing conclusions from his experiments; and rarely concludes too much."[26]

Specific areas of research that Boyle had investigated were also extended into the eighteenth century, and again, in these more focused investigations those who figure prominently often display considerable familiarity with Boyle's writings and research proposals. The area of environmental medicine provides several examples. Boyle's effluvial ideas were found useful in explaining epidemics where no direct contact between infected individuals could be ascertained. His notions about the air as a heterogeneous conglomerate of particles prompted a shift from the traditional ideas that air was one of the non-naturals (influences external to the body that could prompt disease) to the view that air was a primary agent of disease (particles in the air insinuating themselves within the body to directly cause disease). His suggestions about the utility of observing local weather conditions also were followed up in the eighteenth century. These observations furnished a considerable amount of data for physicians. In addition, Boyle's speculations on the local environmental causes of disease encouraged thinking on how such conditions could be modified. This emphasis on prevention had not been part of Hippocratic perspective and was to become an important focus of Enlightenment ideas on public health.

According to James Riley, Boyle made significant contributions to environmental medicine in two broad areas. First, his investigations of the properties of the atmosphere led to "the assumption that decomposition of the properties of the air must contribute to understanding of the diseases caused, transmitted, or influenced by it." Second, his corpuscular philosophy itself, by postulating chemically distinct particles as agents of diseases, "furnished environmentalism with something concrete—albeit still largely hypothetical—to investigate."[27]

Several innovative eighteenth-century investigators made environmental medicine a focus of their work. The best-known probably is the Italian Bernardino Ramazzini, whose *De morbis artificium diatriba* (1700) is considered the pioneer work on occupational diseases. Ramazzini's writing shows that he was clearly familiar with Boyle's ideas.

The work of John Arbuthnot, now better known as a satirist than as a physician, represents an attempt to provide a general theory of environmentalism and to describe a method for obtaining information. His major work in this regard is his *Essay Concerning the Effects of Air on Human Bodies* (1733). Although it does not suggest anything really new, the work is significant for clarifying the main ideas behind environmental medicine.

Arbuthnot was well versed on the work of Boyle, Sydenham, and others who had discussed the role of the atmosphere in disease. For Arbuthnot the starting point was not epidemics, as it had been for Sydenham, but rather the atmosphere itself. Arbuthnot's goal was to collect, quantify, and consolidate information regarding local environmental conditions and *then* to correlate this information with the presence of epidemic diseases. Following Boyle, he discussed the importance of atmospheric pressure, air density, and fluidity as properties of the air that determined how and to what degree atmospheric particles could insinuate themselves into the pores of the body to produce sensible changes. It was the effluvial emanations characteristic of a given local area, combined with these changing atmospheric properties, that explained the rise and fall of epidemics in a particular region. He maintained, therefore, that it was important to conduct chemical analyses of effluvial emanations in addition to collecting local weather data. He emphasized the importance of making careful measurements of temperature, humidity, and atmospheric pressure, which gives his work a more quantitative focus than that of others in England who wrote on this subject at this time.

Although Arbuthnot attempted to provide a blueprint for methodical investigation of environmental conditions, in general, a qualitative approach was preferred by English investigators. For example, Thomas Short, of Sheffield, who made copious notes on weather and the air for nearly twenty years, focused on the variety of factors that could influence disease. As Riley notes, because of the sheer number of the variables he listed, and the impossibility of quantifying these in any meaningful way, English environmental medicine never moved much beyond qualitative description.[28] One of the main criticisms directed against Boyle—that his medical outlook was too broad-based to provide practical guidelines for medical practice—is also applicable to Short.

Eighteenth-century investigations into specific environmental causes of disease did not provide the extensive medical breakthroughs that had been anticipated. No definitive therapeutic ideas evolved out of the work, and progress was hampered by the fact that the basic theory that environmental factors caused disease could never be "proven," given the state of science at that time. However, the intellectual excursions into the theory provided a common ground where natural philosophers and physicians could discuss results of their research—much in the manner Boyle had envisioned. In addition, as Riley notes, Enlightenment notions of improving society and redressing human problems "both inspired and drew inspiration from environmentalism."[29] During the eighteenth-century Enlightenment a considerable literature developed on the subjects of hygiene and public health, which were often tied to right living and moral virtue.[30] The idea that action could be taken to protect the environment from being polluted in the first place (as opposed to neutralizing disease agents once they were present) was to have a much more positive impact on medicine. In this area at least, Boyle's insistence that health was integrally related to environmental conditions and that therefore the environment should be carefully studied proved valuable to medicine.

Boyle's work dealing with the composition of mineral waters was also utilized by later writers. The general scheme for analyzing mineral waters chemically that Boyle had developed in the 1680s provided guidelines for future investigations. However, the lack of an agreed-upon chemical terminology hampered the ability to critique adequately the findings obtained as the result of these investigations. Eighteenth-century work on mineral waters tended to concentrate on the "spiritous" or gaseous components of the waters. Peter Shaw, whose idiosyncratic 1725 edition of Boyle's works was widely read in the eighteenth century, composed a treatise on the Scarborough spa waters in 1734.[31] In it he argued, among other things, that elusive aerial substances might be fixed in mineral waters and that this might account for their medicinal properties.[32] There were also attempts to isolate sediments obtained by evaporation. Both Friedrich Hoffmann and Thomas Short performed investigations of this type; however, they came up with conflicting results.

The eighteenth century saw the development of pneumatic chemistry, which built upon the experimental foundations Boyle had laid. The medical dimensions of pneumatic chemistry included not only identification of gaseous components of the atmosphere and mineral waters that could affect health and disease but also attempts to discover how "vitiated" air could be restored to a more sanative state. Joseph Priestley's experiments in the second half of the eighteenth century included investigations of how common air was naturally corrupted by putrefaction or consumption by fire and how it could be improved, for example, by the purifying action of green plants under the influence of light.[33] Using his pneumatic trough to collect gases over water, Priestley had been able to obtain nitrogen ("phlogisticated air") and nitrogen compounds. In 1772 he devised a method of measuring the "goodness" of the air by mixing common air and nitric oxide ("nitrous air") over water and noting how much the volume of common air diminished.[34] The greater the degree of absorption by nitrous air, the less respirable it became. Equating "respirability" with "goodness," Priestley maintained that one could use this nitrous air test to determine air quality.[35] He believed that such a test would have public health ramifications, providing a means to assess the atmospheric environment of a region. He hoped that ultimately ways of restoring respirable air could be developed. In this way, human society itself would be able to control its environment and improve the quality of life. Such notions spurred the development of "eudiometry" as a technology in the 1770s and became linked with more general ideas of civil and moral reform, as Simon Schaffer has pointed out.[36] Work of this type was consistent with Boyle's original vision that a better understanding of the air would prove useful in improving the human condition.

Boyle's Legacy Assessed

It is evident that many of the ideas that were prominent in Boyle's thought were taken up by later medical writers. Many credited him directly or gave him general praise for his experimental acumen, his modest and conciliatory demeanor, and his interest in seeking ways to improve science and medicine. Certainly, his reputation was sound, and his works were widely read. He had a broad network of associates, and his varied interests (as well as his gentle personality) endeared him to intellectuals of quite differing viewpoints. His various ideas relating to medical theory and practice appear to have been rather well disseminated and to have provided useful suggestions for later medical inquiry.

Nonetheless, Boyle was always perceived more as a cheerleader than as a real guide in efforts to improve medical theory and practice. In part this was because of his lack of formal medical training, but it was also because of the daunting scope of investigations he thought necessary for medical improvement, the inherent disparities between his methodology and the specific needs of the practicing physician, the obscuring effect of Newtonianism, and the extremely tentative and cautious way he forwarded his views.

In the first place, Boyle's focus was so broad that it was considered too general a base on which to build a body of useful knowledge for medical practice. His belief that physicians would know how to evaluate new ideas and adequately discriminate between information that was relevant to their discipline and information that was not relevant was not wholly realistic. In addition, Boyle had not given sufficient attention to the sociological dimensions of the problems medical practitioners were facing at the time he wrote. The reasons why strong collaboration between medical professionals and virtuosi was seen as a threat to professionalism were discussed earlier in this chapter. With the Royal College of Physicians institutionally weak and the number of unlicensed competitors growing, university-trained physicians were being asked both to defend their traditional professional status and to accommodate new ideas. Boyle did not fully appreciate how overwhelming this effort could be. At stake was the fundamental perception of the profession, as Harold Cook has clearly pointed out:

> The consequent debates among physicians therefore grappled with questions about the intellectual foundations upon which their profession ought to rest, and hence about what kind of a profession it would be. To suggest that the medical debates in the period of the "Scientific Revolution" were

merely about physiology or curative techniques *misses the central problem* facing physicians in the period. It distorts our view about the kind of learning upon which the physicians' reputations rested.[37]

Boyle assumed that the gradual incorporation of new knowledge could reform the medical discipline without seriously undermining the status quo of medical professionalism. He did not wish to see the existing social hierarchy altered to the point where formally educated physicians held no higher status than empirics. However, he did not realize how quickly the incorporation of particular bits of information of value to physiology and therapy could threaten the basis of medical education itself—the education foundation that gave the university-trained physician his professional identification in the first place. Galen's *methodus medendi,* the basis of the traditional university curriculum, was vulnerable in that it could not be an object of change and still maintain its utility.[38] By asking that it be the object of change, Boyle left professional physicians adrift. As we have seen, they became aware of this and withdrew from broad identification with the "new science" by 1668.

Many physicians came to believe that they could best serve the future of medicine by lowering their sights and limiting their investigations to the realm of the observed only. A narrower intellectual focus would free physicians from the necessity of suggesting basic causal explanations (even those couched in the "probabilistic" terms Boyle preferred) and allow them to concentrate more directly on investigations of immediate utility, such as specific disease symptoms and classification.

Medical investigators in the eighteenth century in general began to delineate what they considered the proper boundaries for research. Boyle's approach, by contrast, seemed too broad to address physicians' practical, everyday needs. To be fair, Boyle also believed that empirical investigation would yield immediately useful knowledge for physicians and encouraged them to recognize the value of intermediate hypotheses. However, he insisted that physicians search for some more general hypotheses, for this would eventually provide a comprehensive rationale to inform all of their actions. Many physicians chose to ignore this wider search in favor of using observed data as the basis for organizing medical facts into more and more detailed categories. By such an approach, pressure to alter the traditional *methodus medendi* (and revamp the basic medical curriculum) could be reduced, though not stopped. Also, the physician could spend his time more efficiently, focusing on areas of immediate benefit to his practice.

Thus we find many physicians of the late seventeenth and early eighteenth centuries classifying diseases on the basis of clinical observation and deliberately *not* hypothesizing about causes. Erwin Ackerknecht noted that this effort itself created confusions, resulting in a classification mania that "multiplied artificial disease units to the point of absurdity."[39] Yet behind this emphasis on classification was a conscious awareness of the limitations to knowledge of ultimate causes, which made the physician realize that he must relegate his efforts to the realm of the directly observable.

It was not only professional competition and philosophical arguments about the extent of the knowable that turned eighteenth-century medical investigators away from Boyle's suggestions that medical inquiry be broad-based and toward more immediately practical investigations. Patient attitudes also played a role. N. D. Jewson has maintained that patients in the eighteenth century had become so knowledgeable about medical matters that medical discourse was now in the public domain. A physician wishing to establish a reputation could not compete in the medical marketplace unless he had a rationale for treatment that he could convey to the general public in terms they would understand.[40]

The need for physicians to establish credibility in the eyes of their patients also made them focus their energies on developing concepts with clearly delimited parameters. By doing so, they could claim areas of mastery that could be recognized by the laymen as indicators of competency. Malcolm Nicolson suggests that the eighteenth-century physician found in the concept of the metastatic theory of pathogenesis the opportunity to display distinctive mastery of his discipline.[41]

The theory of metastasis is based on the premise that morbific particles of disease in the body move from site to site, prompting different symptoms. The physician gained the confidence of his patient by being able to predict successfully where the morbid matter would transfer and what symptoms the patient would develop. (This same emphasis on prognosis had been the basis of Hippocratic medicine and had provided Greek physicians, who traveled from town to town in search of patients, opportunities to establish their own reputations in the face of constant competition.) What was needed to perform prognosis well was an agreed-upon classification of diseases and observation of characteristic symptoms over the course of illness. This was a confined and limited investigative process, and here again no clear determination of the cause of disease was required. Specialized, not broad-based, research was what was necessary.

It is interesting that the eighteenth-century concept of metastasis itself assumes a corpuscular view of nature and the postulation of qualitatively distinct morbific particles, both of which were central to Boyle's medical thought. Further, Boyle's views of disease included the idea that morbific matter can move through the body and produce localized symptoms. Those eighteenth-century physicians interested in metastasis may have rejected Boyle's broad-based research methodology, but they by no means rejected his theoretical constructs.

If practical necessity and the desire to avoid hypothesizing about the unknowable led physicians away from Boyle's broad-based, open-ended method to a more limited and systematized approach, others were led away by the lure of Newtonianism. Newton's achievement of a mathematical synthesis of terrestrial and celestial operations through his postulation of a universal gravitational force set a standard for scientific inquiry far into the next century.

Newtonian mechanics, buoyed by the certainty of mathematics, conveyed the hope that all natural phenomena could be described in simple and quantitative terms. As Anita Guerrini has indicated, this resulted in efforts to create for the microcosm a set of universal laws similar to those Newton had assigned to the macrocosm.[42] Until the full scope of Newton's matter theory had been articulated and absorbed by his medical followers, however, much of the writing of "Newtonian physicians," such as George Cheyne and Archibald Pitcairne, contained more conventional mechanistic explanations. Cheyne's 1705 work *Philosophical Principles of Natural Religion,* for example, utilized both Boyle's ideas on the structure of matter and his explanation for the elastic quality of the air in terms of "springy particles."[43]

After the success of the *Principia,* Newton's scientific stature grew in an unparalleled way. To espouse a "Newtonian" perspective was to place oneself in the vanguard of scientific "progress." Newton's patronage could make a career. Newton himself was also quite capable of manipulating people to ensure that his philosophical views became dominant.[44]

Although there were significant points of identity between Boyle's and Newton's ideas, especially in the years prior to Newton's publication of his ether theory, there was a tendency on the part of those utilizing or extending the ideas of either man to label them all "Newtonian." This was probably most often the case in the area of Boyle's notions of the hierarchical structure of matter, which Newton had adopted.[45] In other ways, however, Newton's thought encouraged researchers to look in new directions, ultimately giving "Newtonian" medicine a focus distinct from that advocated by Boyle.

First, Newton's followers strongly advocated the use of mathematics and quantification in investigating natural phenomena, including organic phenomena. Although this position was given more lip service than implementation in the biological sciences, it does represent a shift away from

Boyle's highly qualitative methods. Second, Newton's interest in attractive forces operating at the submacroscopic level afforded a conceptualization of physiological processes that Boyle's more standard mechanical views had not provided. Finally, when the second edition of the *Principia* revealed Newton's revived interest in the ether theory, "Newtonian" medical writers attempted to move in this new direction, abandoning explanations that concentrated on the particles themselves for explanations that centered on the medium (the ether) in which these particles moved.[46]

In general, then, we find in the early eighteenth century a conscious attempt by many interested in medical theory to visualize the body as a complex system managed by attractive forces. These Newtonian views in medicine developed gradually:

> The first generation of Newtonians saw in Newton's system of nature a mechanical philosophy with attractions added to tighten things up a bit in areas where mechanisms were obviously inadequate. They did not recognize that his philosophy implied a fundamental restructuring of the entire scientific enterprise. They simply replaced the language of the mechanical philosophy with another; the Newtonian idiom replaced the language of mechanisms. The Newtonians continued to use mechanistic schemes; they simply expressed them differently. They praised the use of mathematics and demonstrated their prowess in that science, but they seldom used quantification or mathematical proof in any meaningful way. They arranged their treatises in axioms and propositions, but . . . gave no indication of logical development along the lines indicated by the mathematical method. Pitcairne [Archibald Pitcairne (1652–1713), a Scottish physician who attempted to base all medical practice upon mechanical principles] came closest to imitating Newton's method . . . but realized . . . that he could therefore make few positive statements concerning the structure of matter. The younger members of the group were far more sanguine; once they had translated conventional physiology and chemistry into Newtonian terms, they felt that they had achieved their goal of a Newtonian cosmos.[47]

The result of this particular trend was that Boyle's own views were overlooked in favor of one promising greater precision and the potential to discover a set of universal, simple laws for the functioning of the human body that paralleled those Newton had discovered as operative in the macrocosm. Newton's vision of how the world operated prompted debates over the nature of matter and the locus of force and shifted attention away from the concepts of particles and pressure differentials, which Boyle had emphasized, to a concept of attractive and repulsive forces.

Boyle's Legacy

Force was seen as nonmechanical but natural. Its cause was unknown. Whether force was intrinsic or extrinsic to matter became a major subject for eighteenth-century debate. Closely related was the question whether matter was inherently active or purely passive. Such questions were of particular interest to anyone investigating the life sciences, and therefore we find the attention of eighteenth-century medical thinkers being drawn to discussions of the role of the soul and the appropriateness of applying machine analogies to the human body.

Boyle, meanwhile, had come to be perceived as more of a traditional "mechanist" than he really was. Clericuzio has pointed out that in the early eighteenth century, Continental writers such as Gottfried Wilhelm Leibniz, who disliked the "occult" implications of Newton's theory of attractive and repulsive forces, began to see Boyle as a truer mechanist than Newton.[48] Peter Shaw, whose edition of Boyle's work was widely read in the eighteenth century, also was a stanch Newtonian, and because of the lack of any truly definitive edition of Boyle's works, Shaw's idiosyncratic interpretation of Boyle was not challenged. The Boyle that many eighteenth-century readers came to know was one seen through Newtonian eyes.

Although nonmechanical agents did play a role in Boyle's philosophy, giving his work a greater flexibility than it would have had if he had taken a strict mechanistic approach to nature, eighteenth-century natural philosophers came to perceive Boyle as a traditional mechanist. In the course of the eighteenth century, medical thinkers backed away from strict mechanical interpretations. Boyle, having become more closely associated with such views, was now more likely to be ignored by medical theorists. Those elements of his thought that they did incorporate, such as his vision of the body as a hydraulico-pneumatic system, were now frequently identified with Newton.

A final explanation why Boyle's message tended to become eclipsed may be that the cautious, tentative way in which Boyle forwarded his suggestions for the improvement of medicine was disconcerting to many of his contemporaries. Boyle's nonconfrontational demeanor (in person and in print) was legendary. Although this may have ensured a wide audience for his views, it caused his contemporaries to view Boyle as not committing himself firmly enough to any position. Boyle, of course, insisted that even probabilistic knowledge was usable, but this message would have been easily lost on contemporaries, especially practicing physicians, who were seeking more solid theories on which to base their professional reputation. Faced with such a proliferation of ideas as occurred in the seventeenth century, the scientific community turned increasingly toward condensation of information and its organization into systems implying a greater degree of certainty than Boyle would have acknowledged.

Boyle's extreme tentativeness was evidently a sore point even when he was at the height of his popularity, as is evident from two letters exchanged between Christian Huygens and Leibniz at the time of his death. In the first, written the day before Boyle died, Huygens bemoans Boyle's reticence to theorize, arguing that it is wrong to hold back from such speculation and wait for certainty.

> Je m'etonnerois si M. Boyle qui a tant de belles experiences, ne seroit arrivé à quelque théorie sur la Chymie, apres y avoir tant medité. Cependant dans ses livres et pour toutes consequences qu'il tire de ses observations, il ne conclut que ce que nous scavons tous scavoir, que tout se fait mecaniquement. Il est peut-être trop reservé. Les hommes excellens nous doivent laisser jusqu'à leur conjectures, et ils ont tort, s'ils ne veuillent donner que des verités certaines.[49]

A few months later, Huygens replied:

> M. Boyle est mort, comme vous scaurez desia sans doute. Il paroit assez etrange qu'il n'ait rien basti sur tant d'experiences dont ses livres sont pleins; mais la chose est difficile, et je ne l'ay jamais cru capable d'une aussi grande application qu'il fait pour establir des principes vraisemblables. Il a bien fait cependant en contredisant à ceux des Chymistes.[50]

For the reasons given above, including the trend toward focusing only on observables, the popularity of Newton and debates over the nature of forces, and the professional need to establish rationales for medical practice that were less overtly tentative, Boyle's views on the improvement of medicine received only mixed attention. In some areas, such as environmental medicine and the theory of metastasis, Boyle's specific influence can be identified. In other areas, Boyle's message seems to have been ignored or obscured. Given the needs of the medical profession, the limited knowledge of chemistry at the time, and the dominance of a Newtonian perspective suggesting that the body's operations should be viewed in terms of the action of quantifiable, short-range forces analogous to gravity, it is understandable why Boyle's qualitative, multifaceted, long-range, investigative methodology was not more popular.

Even if it had been accepted, experimental methods in the sciences had not yet sufficiently developed to produce many solid findings. Despite his insistence on the value of chemical analysis for understanding nature, Boyle himself had no clear notion of what constituted a chemical element. In fact, in his anxiety to distinguish his methodology from that of the Aristotelians, he deliberately denied postulating specific elements, depending rather upon the idea that any substance should be considered elemental only temporarily and arbitrarily, until analytical techniques had been sufficiently perfected to break it down further. His efforts to pin down precise chemical entities were also hampered by his postulation that all matter was essentially transmutable. Although Boyle did believe that ultimately only a limited number of primary substances existed in nature, he was not yet able to identify any of them.[51] Such a concept would have rendered little service to physicians seeking to define the causes of disease in precise chemical terms.

In addition, Boyle's method of validating findings by collective consensus rather than controlled rigorous experiment was too subjective. Perhaps the greatest shortcoming in Boyle's experimental program was his failure to base it on the use of the "crucial experiment," whereby, by systematically eliminating all variables save one, one could reach more objective conclusions. Boyle's determination to emphasize the collaborative aspect of scientific activity is certainly understandable. He found unethical the secrecy and self-promotion that had so characterized chemistry, and often empirical medicine as well, in his day. Growing up in England during the difficult years of religious upheaval and extremist sectarianism, Boyle came to abhor anything suggestive of religious enthusiasm. Scientific knowledge would increase as the result of the hard work of moral individuals, for this was God's intention; it would not emerge full-blown from the sudden spiritual illumination of a few adepts. Because his religious views (not to mention his views of social propriety) were so interwoven into his scientific thought, Boyle's attention often was focused more on the conduct of the experimenters than on the conduct of the experiment.

Because he was anxious to acquire vast amounts of information—too vast, in fact, for him to test firsthand—Boyle's perspective was generally too inclusivist. True experimental rigor would have required a more discriminating attitude toward experimental evidence, yet his modesty and conscious eclecticism prevented him from adopting a more judgmental posture. This prevented him from "weeding out" any idea that could not be conclusively disproved. The result was an unwieldy conglomeration of "probable facts" that confused rather than illuminated thinking about nature.

Finally, Boyle's use of analogy to bridge the realms of the observed and the unobserved can be seen as problematic. Given the limited state of experimental science in his age, analogy was probably one of the few available techniques open to one who eschewed a priori reasoning about causes. However, such an approach had its limitations. especially in dealing with such complex matters as physiological function.

"Divulging of Useful Truths in Physick"

How, then, are we to judge Boyle's relevance to medical thought? Living in much simpler times, before the era of scientific specialization, before adequate instrumentation, and at a time when experimental procedure was in its infancy, Boyle posited a set of ideas that he thought would lead to progress in medicine. He held that natural phenomena could be analyzed in chemical and mechanical terms, despite the fact that such an approach in his day could only render speculative conclusions. He grappled with the notions of chemical change before chemistry had been established as a quantitative science with a consistent terminology and before even he could articulate clearly the notion of a chemical element. He offered a procedural method that relied on the accumulation of knowledge over time, knowledge built up by hypotheses, but never itself certain. In an age in which ancient authority was still relied on, he boldly affirmed the legitimacy of fresh discovery. He empowered physicians with notions that the broadest understanding of nature could best inform their actions and that they need not restrict their therapeutic decisions to those dictated by any single set of theoretical constructs. His emphasis on experiment as a primary investigative tool and the conviction that scientific knowledge could be extended through the efforts of many men working together led to a new awareness of the potential of science for the quality of life. Later investigators were to take up this theme and to develop it in much more sophisticated ways, providing methods and procedures that had tangible results for both individual and public health. Specific areas of his thought, such as the role of the environment and the air on human health, did provide inspiration for later work. If Boyle made no specific medical discovery that led to the cure of a disease or the institution of any novel mode of therapy, nonetheless, through his words and his own example, he instilled in his contemporaries and in his successors as well an optimism that discoveries of great moment could be achieved. For the physician as for all other men, this was a most profound legacy.

NOTES

Introduction

1. It is important to note that the formal term *methodus medendi* refers not to rules of technical procedure but to a logical mode of investigation, a means of ensuring that one's conclusions were sound. Galen's *methodus medendi* primarily involved synthesizing information obtained from a rational analysis of what constituted the state of health. By the seventeenth century, some of the basic features of Galen's *methodus* were coming under attack, leading many to seek an alternative logical base. See Jeffrey Boss, "The 'Methodus Medendi' as an Index of Change in the Philosophy of Medical Science in the Sixteenth and Seventeenth Centuries," *History and Philosophy of the Life Sciences* 1 (1979): 13–42.

2. *Experimenta et Observationes Physicae,* in *The Works of the Honorable Robert Boyle,* ed. Thomas Birch, 6 vols. (1772; reprint, Hildesheim: Georg Olms, 1966), 5:583; hereinafter cited as *Works.*

3. The English legal year used to begin on 25 March. After the shift to the present calendar, it became customary to give the year according to both the old and the new calendar for dates between 1 January and 25 March, in order to avoid confusion.

4. Henry Oldenburg, Commonplace Book, 1660, Royal Society of London, MS. 1; hereinafter Royal Society manuscripts will be abbreviated as RS MS. Marie Boas [Hall] dates this "Essay of Turning Poisons into Medicines" at about 1650 (see *Robert Boyle and Seventeenth-Century Chemistry* [Cambridge: Cambridge University Press, 1958], 29).

5. *Usefulness of Experimental Natural Philosophy, Works,* 2:85–87. In the excerpt, Boyle discusses whether vipers should be properly classified as poisons and provides a remedy for viper bites.

6. John F. Fulton, *A Bibliography of the Honorable Robert Boyle,* 2d ed. (Oxford: Clarendon Press, 1961), 118.

Chapter 1 The Formative Years

1. For an in-depth description of Richard Boyle's rise to fame and his personal ethics see Nicholas Canny, *The Upstart Earl: A Study of the Social and Mental World of Richard Boyle, First Earl of Cork: 1566–1643* (Cambridge: Cambridge University Press, 1982).

2. Ibid., 147; James R. Jacob, *Robert Boyle and the English Revolution: A Study in Social and Intellectual Change* (New York: Burt Franklin, 1977), 25–27.

3. Jacob, *Boyle and the English Revolution,* 26.

4. This autobiographical fragment, "An Account of Philaretus during his Mi-

nority," is reproduced in R. E. W. Maddison, *The Life of the Honourable Robert Boyle* (New York: Barnes & Noble, 1969), 2–45. Maddison provides evidence to suggest that it was written between January 1648 and July 1649.

5. Ibid., 22.

6. Jacob suggests that while Boyle was in Geneva he had considerable contact with Jean Diodati, an irenic preacher of the Swiss Reformed Church and a friend and colleague of Henry Wotton's, who resided there then. Jacob sees Diodati as another early source of Boyle's interest in irenical Protestantism (Jacob, *Boyle and the English Revolution,* 26–27).

7. Robert Boyle to Isaac Marcombes, 22 October 1646, *Works,* 1:xxxiii. The circumstances of Boyle's arrest are unknown, but that it occurred is not surprising, given the prominence of his family and the fact that other family members were vocal supporters of one or the other side of the conflict. (While Lady Ranelagh herself was a strong supporter of the parliamentary cause, Boyle's brother Roger, Baron Broghill, was at this time a staunch Royalist.)

8. The development of Boyle's ethics has been investigated by both Jacob and, more recently, John T. Harwood (*The Early Essays and Ethics of Robert Boyle,* ed. Harwood [Carbondale: Southern Illinois University Press, 1991]). Although Harwood and Jacob differ on the inspiration for Boyle's ethical views, both admit that a strong providentialism underlies his ideas on moral behavior.

9. "Account of Philaretus," in Maddison, *Life,* 16.

10. Individuals commonly took responsibility for their own ailments in the seventeenth and eighteenth centuries. See Dorothy Porter and Roy Porter, *Patients' Progress: Doctors and Doctoring in Eighteenth Century England* (Stanford, Calif.: Stanford University Press, 1989), 35–53, on the prevalence of self-medication, distrust of doctors, and hypochondria among Englishmen in this age.

11. Harwood, *Early Essays,* xlv.

12. Although the subject has been analyzed most fully by Jacob and Harwood, other modern writers have also addressed it. See, e.g., H. Fisch, "The Scientist as Priest: A Note on Robert Boyle's Natural Theology," *Isis* 15 (1953): 252–65, and extensive comments in Richard S. Westfall, *Science and Religion in Seventeenth-Century England* (Ann Arbor: University of Michigan Press, 1973), and Michael Hunter, *Science and Society in Restoration England* (Cambridge: Cambridge University Press, 1981).

13. The fragment is found in RS MS. 195. Jacob notes that another Royal Society manuscript, MS. 192, entitled "The Ethicall Elements," appears to be a draft of the first portion of MS. 195 (Jacob, *Boyle and the English Revolution,* 191 n. 6).

14. "Materialls & Addenda Design'd towards the Structure & compleating of Treatises already begun or Written. January the 25th 1649/50," Boyle Papers, vol. 36, Royal Society of London; hereinafter the Boyle Papers will be cited as BP.

15. Boyle to Lady Ranelagh, 2 August 1649, *Works,* 6:48.

16. Boyle to [John Mallet], November 1651, B.M. Harl. MS. 7003, fol. 179, quoted in Maddison, *Life,* 78.

17. Boyle to Lady Ranelagh, 6 March 1646/47, *Works,* 1:xxvi.

18. BP 28.

Notes to Pages 11–15

19. "An Epistolical Discourse of Philaretus to Empericus, inviting all true lovers of Vertue and Mankind, to a free and generous Communication of their Secrets and Receipts in Physick," in *Chymical, Medicinal, and Chyrurgical Addresses made to S. Hartlib* (London 1655). Boyle informed Hartlib in a letter of 8 May 1647 (*Works,* 1:xli) that he had completed this treatise.

20. The well-known work of Thomas K. Merton, *Science, Technology, and Society in Seventeenth Century England* (New York: Harper & Row, 1970), linking Puritan sensitivities to scientific enterprise, was first published as a monograph in *Osiris* 4 (1938): 360–632. This view has not lacked for supporters or critics, even though, as Steven Shapin has pointed out, Merton himself was far from dogmatic in his presentation (Steven Shapin, "Understanding the Merton Thesis," *Isis* 79 [1988]: 594–605). Since Merton, many other scholars have attempted to analyze the role of identifiable religious groups in the advancement of science. These include Barbara J. Shapiro ("Latitudinarianism and Science in Seventeenth Century England," in *The Intellectual Revolution of the Seventeenth Century,* ed. Charles Webster [London: Routledge & Kegan Paul, 1974], 286–316); Charles Webster (*The Great Instauration: Science, Medicine, and Reform, 1626–1660* [New York: Holmes & Meier, 1975]); James R. Jacob *(Boyle and the English Revolution);* and Lotte Mulligan and Glenn Mulligan ("Reconstructing Restoration Science," *Social Studies of Science* 11 [1981]: 327–64). Nevertheless, no consensus has been reached, and the debate continues as strong as ever.

21. Peter Elmer has suggested that irenicism was the spur to the widespread interest in new forms of medical practice and theory in mid-seventeenth-century England (see his "Medicine, Religion, and the Puritan Revolution," in *The Medical Revolution of the Seventeenth Century,* ed. Roger French and Andrew Wear [Cambridge: Cambridge University Press, 1989], 45).

22. For more on this see H. R. Trevor-Roper, "Three Foreigners and the Philosophy of the English Revolution," *Encounter* 14 (1960): 3–20. The advent of the Irish Rebellion and political deterioration into civil war thwarted any implementation of these plans. Hartlib, however, spent the following years promoting his cause, and he continued to gather around him men eager to carry out his and their own specific projects for the betterment of society.

23. *A Description of the Famous Kingdome of Macaria* (London, 1641). The work is reproduced in Charles Webster, *Samuel Hartlib and the Advancement of Learning* (Cambridge: Cambridge University Press, 1970).

24. Webster notes that Comenius was considerably influenced by Bacon (see Webster, *Hartlib,* 22).

25. This argument is used by Charles Webster in "New Light on the Invisible College: The Social Relations of English Science in the Mid-Seventeenth Century," *Transactions of the Royal Historical Society* 24 (1974): 19–42. Canny reiterates Webster's argument (*Upstart Earl,* 143).

26. This letter is cited in G. H. Turnbull, *Hartlib, Dury, and Comenius: Gleanings from Hartlib's Papers* (Liverpool: Liverpool University Press, 1947), 27–28.

27. Harwood, *Early Essays,* xliv.

Notes to Pages 16–19

28. Canny argues that Boyle's father instilled his values, including his irenical perspective and his sense of social order, in all of his children, structuring their education carefully to inculcate these values. Lady Ranelagh and Robert Boyle certainly shared similar attitudes toward spiritual reform, which might be traced to the influence of Richard Boyle. However, it should also be noted that Richard Boyle deliberately limited personal contact with his sons, insisting that they be raised apart from him, and that Robert specifically spent "mere months" with his father before his death (Canny, *Upstart Earl,* 98–104).

29. *Macaria,* in Webster, *Hartlib,* 83.

30. That Boyle was seriously troubled by the ethical and moral component of his alchemical interests has recently been discussed by Michael Hunter in "Alchemy, Magic, and Moralism in the Thought of Robert Boyle," *British Journal for the History of Science* 23 (1990): 387–410.

31. Webster, *Great Instauration,* 70.

32. Boyle to Marcombes, 22 October 1646, *Works,* 1:xxxiv.

33. Boyle to Francis Tallents, 20 February 1647, ibid., 1:xxxiv–xxxv.

34. The only extant letters in which Boyle refers specifically to the Invisible College are the letters to Marcombes and Tallents cited above and a letter to Samuel Hartlib dated 8 May 1647 (ibid., 1:xl). Whether several other Boyle letters from this period that mention "colleges" or "philosophical colleges" refer to the Invisible College specifically is still a debating point for scholars.

35. Ibid., 1:xlii. For opposing arguments see discussions in Maddison, *Life,* 68–70; Webster, *Great Instauration,* 57–58; and idem, "New Light," 21–23. The arguments against identifying the Invisible College with the Gresham Group center on the lack of any reference to Boyle in Wallis's or Sprat's accounts of the origins of the Royal Society, on the apparent emphasis of the Gresham Group on pure science rather than its practical applications, and on the fact that Boyle was unknown to the leaders of the Gresham Group until 1653.

36. On the view associating the Invisible College with members of the Hartlib circle see discussions in Boas, *Robert Boyle and Seventeenth-Century Chemistry;* Margery Purver, *The Royal Society: Concept and Creation* (Cambridge: MIT Press, 1967); R. H. Syfret, "The Origins of the Royal Society," *Notes and Records of the Royal Society of London* 5 (1948): 75–137; and Francis A. Yates, *The Rosicrucian Enlightenment* (London: Routledge & Kegan Paul, 1972). On challenges to this view see G. H. Turnbull, "Samuel Hartlib's Influence on the Early History of the Royal Society," *Notes and Records of the Royal Society of London* 10 (1953): 101–30; Webster, "New Light," 23–25; and Canny, *Upstart Earl,* 139–50.

37. Carolyn Merchant, *The Death of Nature: Women, Ecology, and the Scientific Revolution* (New York: Harper & Row, 1980).

38. For a discussion of this work, along with a transcription and commentary, see Margaret E. Rowbottom, "The Earliest Published Writing of Robert Boyle," *Annals of Science* 6 (1948–50): 376–89.

39. Boyle to Lady Ranelagh, 31 August 1649, *Works,* 6:49–50.

40. The first national pharmacopoeia, the *Pharmacopoeia Londinensis,* issued in 1618, had included chemical remedies along with the traditional Galenic ones,

despite the difficulties of accounting for their effectiveness in terms of Galenic notions of humoral equilibrium. For fuller discussion of the history of Paracelsian ideas in England see Allen G. Debus, *The English Paracelsians* (New York: Neale Watson, 1965). For comments on the shift of focus in the late 1640s see also Webster, *Great Instauration,* 274–76.

41. Men with chemical interests who were closely associated with Hartlib at this time included George Starkey, Frederick Clodius, Robert Child, Frederick Kretschmar, Peter Staehl, Johannes Fortitudo Hartprecht, Johannes Sibertus Kuffeler, Albert Otho Faber, and Johannes Brun (see Charles Webster, "English Medical Reformers of the Puritan Revolution," *Ambix* 14 [1967]: 16–41).

42. BP 25 and 8, respectively.

43. George Starkey and Boyle had worked to develop this remedy sometime in 1651 or 1652 (see John J. O'Brien, "Samuel Hartlib's Influence on Robert Boyle's Scientific Development. Part I: The Stalbridge Period," *Annals of Science* 21 [1965]: 6).

44. Elmer, "Medicine, Religion, and the Puritan Revolution," 43.

45. BP 8 and 25, fols. 153–56.

46. Marie Boas [Hall], "An Early Version of Boyle's *Sceptical Chymist,*" *Isis* 45 (1954): 153–68.

47. See Hartlib to Boyle, 25 May 1658 and 29 November 1659 (*Works,* 6:109, 136), and Henry Oldenburg to Boyle, 20 March 1660 (ibid., 6:145).

48. Hartlib to Boyle, 14 September 1658, ibid., 6:114.

49. Ibid.

50. See Webster, *Great Instauration,* 260-61.

51. Johann Christian Agricola to Boyle, 6 April 1668, *Works,* 6:650.

52. Frederick Clodius to Boyle, 12 December 1663, BP 2, item 17.

53. Paracelsus held that there were three basic principles (the *tria prima):* salt, representing fixity and incombustibility; sulfur, representing inflammability; and mercury, representing volatility and fusibility.

54. See the full discussion in Elmer, "Medicine, Religion, and the Puritan Revolution," 10–45.

55. Hunter, *Science and Society,* 25.

56. This reference to Boyle as a fellow Helmontian appears in the dedication of Starkey's major work, *Pyrotechny Asserted,* published in 1658. Starkey was recognized by his contemporaries as an avid promoter of Van Helmont.

57. Allen G. Debus, *The Chemical Philosophy: Paracelsian Science and Medicine in the Sixteenth and Seventeenth Centuries,* 2 vols. (New York: Science History Publications, 1977), 2:473–92. In this view, Boyle is seen as following an intellectual path similar to that of Walter Charleton (see also Nina Rattner Gelbart, "The Intellectual Development of Walter Charleton," *Ambix* 18 [1971]: 149–68).

58. The interest of the radical sectaries in occult philosophies (and the desire of moderate Protestants to distance themselves from them) is described in James R. Jacob and Margaret C. Jacob, "The Anglican Origins of Modern Science: The Metaphysical Foundations of the Whig Constitution," *Isis* 71 (1980): 251–67.

59. John Henry, "Occult Qualities and the Experimental Philosophy: Active

Principles in Pre-Newtonian Matter Theory," *History of Science* 24 (1986): 371 n. 19.

60. Jacob, *Boyle and the English Revolution,* 112.

61. Hunter, "Alchemy, Magic, and Moralism," 391–92.

62. Vern L. Bullough, *The Development of Medicine as a Profession* (New York: S. Karger, 1966), 108. Bullough explains that the institutionalization of medicine within the medieval university allowed clear professional distinctions to emerge between those in possession of formal medical knowledge (preserved in Latin and imparted as part of a formal, regulated curriculum) and ordinary laymen, for whom such knowledge was much less accessible.

63. Ibid., 109–10.

64. Harold J. Cook, *Decline of the Old Medical Regime in Stuart London* (Ithaca: Cornell University Press, 1986), 20, 22–23.

65. The Royal College could never fully regulate medical practice in London. Enforcement of licensing laws was often inadequate and inconsistent. Even university-trained physicians took exception to the idea that they needed the college's permission to practice in London, since, as Cook notes, "university degrees and licenses in medicine and surgery specified that their holders had the right to practice throughout England" (ibid., 79).

66. Ibid., 72. Even when the college was most powerful, it could not entirely regulate medical practice even in London (ibid., 79).

67. Webster discusses this at length in *Great Instauration,* chap. 4. For a full description of the activities of the Royal College of Physicians in this period see Cook, *Decline.*

68. Cook, *Decline,* 108–9.

69. On the addition of chemical remedies into the national pharmacopoeia see Debus, *English Paracelsians,* 152–55. On the continuing discussion of chemical medicines in the Royal College of Physicians see Cook, *Decline,* 117.

70. Webster, *Great Instauration,* 263–64. For more detail on Biggs's views see Allen Debus, "Paracelsian Medicine: Noah Biggs and the Problem of Medical Reform," in *Medicine in Seventeenth Century England: A Symposium held at UCLA in Honor of C. D. O'Malley,* ed. Debus (Berkeley and Los Angeles: University of California Press, 1974), 34–38.

71. Andrew Cunningham, "Thomas Sydenham: Epidemics, Experiment, and the 'Good Old Cause,'" in French and Wear, *Medical Revolution of the Seventeenth Century,* 170–71.

72. See Jacob, *Boyle and the English Revolution,* 43–82.

73. Boyle's early belief in the usefulness of anatomy shows an additional divergence of his thought from that of the Helmontians, since Van Helmont had rejected the study of anatomy as being of little value to practical medicine.

74. Harvey worked at Oxford from 1642 to 1646, focusing his investigations primarily on embryology.

75. Webster, *Great Instauration,* 142. See also *Dictionary of Scientific Biography,* s.v. "Nathaniel Highmore."

76. Robert G. Frank, Jr., *Harvey and the Oxford Physiologists: A Study of Scien-*

tific Ideas (Berkeley and Los Angeles: University of California Press, 1980), 97–99.

77. There is evidence of a specific agreement between Highmore and Harvey to publish the results of their embryological research (see *Dictionary of Scientific Biography,* s.v. "Nathaniel Highmore." Highmore's work appeared in the same year (1651) as Harvey's *De generatione animalium.*

78. The "powder of sympathy," when applied to a weapon or other object tainted with the victim's blood, was supposed to convey itself (via sympathetic magic) to the wound, affecting healing. "Weapon salve" worked essentially in the same way.

79. Jacob *(Boyle and the English Revolution)* and Hunter *(Science and Society)* both refer to Boyle's concern about engaging only in scientific pursuits that were morally acceptable. His sensitivity about finding religious justification for his *chemical* activities has already been noted above.

80. The extant draft of this treatise, "Of ye Atomicall Philosophy," can be found in BP 26, fols. 162–75. Frank notes that the folio sheets are misbound in this volume (*Harvey and Oxford,* 316 n. 28). Due to this confusion, R. S. Westfall's reprint of this paper, in "Unpublished Boyle Papers Relating to Scientific Method," *Annals of Science* 12 (1956): 63–73, 103–17, includes only the first two leaves.

81. Frank suggests that William Petty (whose work will be discussed below) was probably the most appropriate intermediary to convey these ideas into England, since Petty had studied with the medical Cartesian Cornelis van Hooghelande in Holland and was active in the Hobbesian circle in Paris in the mid-1640s, when Gassendi was in that city (Frank, *Harvey and Oxford,* 92).

82. Boyle Letters, vol. 7, no. 17, Royal Society of London; hereinafter the Boyle Letters will be cited as BL.

83. "Materials & Addenda . . . January the 25th 1649/50," BP 36.

84. Digby's explanation of the sympathetic powder appears first in chapter 18 of the first of Digby's "Two Treatises," "Of Bodies," in 1644 (see Betty Jo Dobbs, "Studies in the Natural Philosophy of Sir Kenelm Digby. Part I," *Ambix* 18 [1971]: 1–25).

85. BP 36. Maddison dates the list in which Boyle refers to this treatise as only slightly later than the list of January 1649/50 (Maddison, *Life,* 76).

86. Nathaniel Highmore, *The History of Generation . . . To which is joyned a Discourse of the Cure of Wounds by Sympathy* (London, 1651), 128–33.

87. Ibid., 4–6 (emphasis added).

88. "Two Essays concerning the Unsuccessfulness of Experiments: Second Essay—Of Unsucceeding Experiments," in *Certain Physiological Essays, Works,* 1:344.

89. William Petty to Boyle, 15 April 1653, ibid., 6:139.

90. *Dictionary of Scientific Biography,* s.v. "Nathaniel Highmore."

91. *Some Motives and Incentives to the Love of God (Seraphick Love), Works,* 1:262.

92. Quoted in Turnbull, "Samuel Hartlib's Influence," 122.

93. Hartlib to Boyle, 9 May 1648, *Works,* 6:77.

Notes to Pages 34–38

94. *Usefulness of Experimental Natural Philosophy,* ibid., 2:7.

95. Ibid., 2:14.

96. Hartlib to Boyle, 16 November 1647, ibid., 6:76.

97. Petty to Boyle, 21 June 1648, ibid., 6:136–37.

98. This plan is described in Webster, *Great Instauration,* 293–96.

99. Ann Green was the victim of a clumsy execution attempt. When her body was brought to the dissecting room, the attending physicians Petty and John Wilkins detected signs of life and revived her. The case created a national sensation.

100. For a general discussion of the Gresham College Group and the relocation of many of its members to Oxford see Douglas McKie, "The Origins and Foundation of the Royal Society of London," *Notes and Records of the Royal Society of London* 15 (1960): 1–37. Information on specific activities of the Oxford Philosophical Club is provided in Robert G. Frank, Jr., "John Aubrey, F.R.S., John Lydall, and Science at Commonwealth Oxford," ibid. 27 (1973): 193–217.

101. Boyle to Clodius, [April 1654,] *Works,* 6:54–55.

102. Petty to Boyle, 15 April 1653, ibid., 6:137–39.

103. John Gascoigne describes how the universities provided a strong sense of collegiality and a solid institutional base for the study of the human body, chemistry, and botany and notes that biomedical advancement occurred almost exclusively in a university context ("A Reappraisal of the Role of the Universities in the Scientific Revolution," in *Reappraisals of the Scientific Revolution,* ed. David C. Lindberg and Robert S. Westman [Cambridge: Cambridge University Press, 1990], 234–34). Boyle's medical interests, his maturing skill as an experimenter, and his commitment to organized, collaborative science would have made the Oxford environment enticing at this time, even more so if Hartlib's circle was fragmented.

104. Jacob and Jacob, "Anglican Origins," 253–54. See also Thomas Gieryn, "Distancing Science from Religion in Seventeenth-Century England," *Isis* 79 (1988): 582–93.

105. BP 37.

106. For example, Henry Oldenburg wrote to congratulate *Boyle* upon the approval by Parliament in 1657 of a proposed scheme for funding Hartlib's Office of Address, which indicates that Boyle was still utilizing his influence to aid Hartlib in his endeavors (Oldenburg to Boyle, 22 September 1657, *Works,* 6:142).

107. Anthony Clericuzio, "A Redefinition of Boyle's Chemistry and Corpuscular Philosophy," *Annals of Science* 47 (1990): 566, 568.

Chapter 2 Developing a Philosophy of Nature

1. For a discussion of the formalization of knowledge gathering and confirmation among seventeenth-century English experimental scientists see Steven Shapin and Simon Schaffer, *Leviathan and the Air-Pump: Hobbes, Boyle, and the Experimental Life* (Princeton: Princeton University Press, 1985); and Steven Shapin, "The House of Experiment in Seventeenth-Century England," *Isis* 79 (1988): 373–404.

2. John Wilkins to Boyle, 6 September 1653, *Works,* 6:633–34.

3. Lady Ranelagh to Boyle, 12 October [1653], ibid., 6:523–24.

4. Frank, *Harvey and Oxford,* 45–46.

5. Birch, "Life of Boyle," in *Works,* 1:liv.

6. Both James and Margaret Jacob and Barbara Shapiro have attempted to describe as latitudinarian the proclivities of a large group of scientific investigators working at Oxford in the 1650s and in London after the Restoration. The Jacobs define as the central tenets of latitudinarianism the "repudiation of predestination, a concomitant emphasis on free will and striving as the keys to salvation, and an almost obsessive concern for design, order, and harmony as the primary manifestations of God's role in the universe" (Jacob and Jacob, "Anglican Origins," 258). Shapiro's more extensive definition of what constituted a latitudinarian position includes: the attempt to find a middle way between skepticism and certainty (leading in science to an emphasis on hypothesis without overt metaphysics); a concern for the moral over the doctrinal aspects of theology; a overall distaste for dogmatism (seen in the scientific attitude of humility before an increasing body of facts); a movement toward natural religion; an emphasis on moderation and a willingness to give way to the judgments of others; the belief that the civil government had authority to set forms of public prayer, to which the individual should comply; and a simplified style of discourse (Shapiro, "Latitudinarianism," 301–2 and passim). Shapiro suggests that much of what Charles Webster has ascribed to the Puritan view of science was actually part of the latitudinarian perspective. Webster, however, has responded that Shapiro has defined latitudinarianism so broadly that it subsumes Puritanism (Webster, *Intellectual Revolution,* 18–20). With regard to Boyle, there are elements of both the Jacobs' and Shapiro's definitions of latitudinarianism that do not seem to apply. To discuss this at length in a book focusing on Boyle's medical thought is not necessarily appropriate; however, it should become evident over the next several chapters that for Boyle, the notion of predestination seems particularly strong, obligation is primary over free will, and although he believed in the right of the civil government to establish forms of public prayer, in his unpublished manuscript "The Plague of London from the Hand of God," written during the plague year of 1665, he makes an impassioned plea on behalf of those who were noncompliant, particularly Quakers (BP 14, item 2, fols. 28r–42v).

7. Hunter, *Science and Society,* 116–17.

8. Works published by Boyle during his sojourn at Oxford include: *Seraphick Love* (written in 1648, published in 1659); *New Experiments, Physico-Mechanical, Touching the Spring of the Air* (written in 1659, published in 1660); *Certain Physiological Essays* (written before 1657, published in 1661); *Sceptical Chymist* (1661); *A Defense of the Doctrine Touching the Spring and Weight of the Air* (1662); *Considerations Touching the Usefulness of Experimental Natural Philosophy, Part I* (written in 1647–49, published in 1663); *Experiments and Considerations Touching Colours* (1664); *Hydrostatical Paradoxes* (written in 1664, published in 1666); *Origin of Forms and Qualities* (1666). Two works published after he moved from Oxford but written during his stay there are *The Usefulness of Experimental Natural Phi-*

losophy, pt. 2 (written ca. 1665, published in 1671), and *The Excellency of Theology* (written in 1665, published in 1674).

9. Louis Trenchard More, *The Life and Works of the Honourable Robert Boyle* (London: Oxford University Press, 1944), 130. One should not assume from More's comments that Boyle became more prolific after his stroke necessitated a more sedentary lifestyle, for some of the work published in this period was written much earlier. Boyle was notorious for not following through on organizing his material or editing it; therefore, frequently treatises published in one decade refer to experiments performed years earlier. Yet it is clear that despite his weakened condition after his stroke, Boyle attempted as best he could to continue his scientific investigations and to keep writing (aided by amanuenses).

10. RS MS. 194, fol. 22r–22v.

11. BP 37, Misc., quoted in A. C. Crombie, *Medieval and Early Modern Science,* 2 vols. (Garden City, N.Y.: Doubleday Anchor Books, 1959), 2:297. There are several different versions of this fragment in Boyle's unpublished papers.

12. Boyle's inspiration for this view is obviously the Baconian inductive method, but Boyle probably perceived more clearly than Bacon that the development of lower-level ("good") hypotheses would take quite some time, so much so that for all intents and purposes scientific work was performed almost exclusively at this "lower" level (of establishing "good" hypotheses), while the development of "excellent" hypotheses was a more distant goal.

13. *Usefulness of Experimental Natural Philosophy, Works,* 2:61.

14. *Discourse of Things above Reason,* ibid., 4:461.

15. Lotte Mulligan, "'Reason,' 'Right Reason,' and 'Revelation' in Mid-Seventeenth Century England," in *Occult and Scientific Mentalities in the Renaissance,* ed. Brian Vickers (Cambridge: Cambridge University Press, 1984), 375–401.

16. Boyle discusses this categorization of "truths" in *Appendix to the First Part of the Christian Virtuoso, Works,* 6:709.

17. *Usefulness of Experimental Natural Philosophy,* ibid., 2:45. The "clockwork metaphor," of course, was by no means original to Boyle. Referring to the observed world as a clock whose internal components were known only to God had by Boyle's time become common among mechanistic philosophers.

18. *Certain Physiological Essays,* ibid., 1:308.

19. Commonplace Book, RS MS. 185, fol. 31, cited in Clericuzio, "Redefinition," 574.

20. That there was indeed an order underlying nature was something that Boyle, of course, believed on theological grounds.

21. Maurice Mandelbaum, *Philosophy, Science, and Sense Perception: Historical and Critical Studies* (Baltimore: Johns Hopkins Press, 1964), 114.

22. "That the Goods of Mankind may be . . . Increased by the Naturalist's Insight into Trades," in *Usefulness of Experimental Natural Philosophy,* pt. 2, *Works,* 3:443.

23. *Some Specimens of an Attempt to make Chymical Experiments useful to . . . the Corpuscular Philosophy,* ibid., 1:358.

24. He argues the validity of this assumption in *Of the Excellency and Grounds*

of the Mechanical Hypothesis, criticizing those who do not accept mechanical explanations of "hidden transactions that pass among the minute particles of bodies" by suggesting that "therefore to say, that tho in natural bodies, whose bulk is manifest and their structure visible, the mechanical principles may be usefully admitted, that are not to be extended to such portions of matter, whose parts and texture are invisible; may perhaps look to some, as if a man should allow, that the laws of mechanism may take place in a town clock, but cannot in a pocket-watch" (ibid., 4:71).

25. See "Essay I, Of the Porousness of Animal Bodies," in *Experiments and Considerations about the Porosity of Bodies,* ibid., 4:768.

26. *Certain Physiological Essays,* ibid., 1:300–301.

27. Boyle explicitly denied that he was a true skeptic, explaining his position by an analogy involving a purse full of guineas, some counterfeit, some adulterated, some good, where his reaction would be not to throw out the whole purse but to select out the good coins and purify others where possible ("Author's Preface," in *Experiments and Notes about the Producibleness of Chymical Principles,* ibid., 1:591). Henry G. Van Leeuwen characterized this position as one of "constructive skepticism," based on "a recognition that the real structure of nature is unknowable and a judicious proportioning of assent to evidence" (*The Problem of Certainty in English Thought, 1630–1690* [The Hague: Martinus Nijhoff, 1963], 105).

28. Henry, "Occult Qualities," 364–65.

29. Boyle refers to Gassendi as "a great favourite of mine" in a letter to Hartlib of 8 May 1647 (*Works,* 1:xli).

30. "History of Particular Qualities," ibid., 3:297-98.

31. The following is a paraphrase of Boyle's description of these principles in ibid.

32. See Clericuzio, "Redefinition," 568–69 and 569 n. 34.

33. This classification was first forwarded in *Origin of Forms and Qualities* and represents a refinement of his earlier views expressed in his treatise "Of ye Atomicall Philosophy."

34. Clericuzio, "Redefinition," 579–83.

35. *Origin of Forms and Qualities, Works,* 3:29. Descartes had also denied that atoms were truly indivisible.

36. Ibid., 30.

37. Clericuzio concludes from this that for Boyle, chemistry is not subordinated to mechanical philosophy, for it is not necessary to reduce all findings to mechanical principles ("Redefinition," 588). Chemical analysis provides those "intermediate theories" that Boyle sees as so useful in science. Here again, we see the value of Boyle's levels of hypothesis. Chemical investigation and mechanistic theorizing exist in tandem with each other. There is no need to choose between a chemical and a mechanical view of nature. All Boyle rejects is the idea that chemical attributes are inherent in uncompounded substances.

38. Ibid., 571.

39. *An Hydrostatical Discourse, Works,* 3:598.

Notes to Pages 55–60

40. *The Christian Virtuoso,* ibid., 5:521.

41. James and Margaret Jacob have suggested (Jacob and Jacob, "Anglican Origins," 259) that corpuscularians rejected Descartes because of his radical separation of spirit and matter, since "the primacy of spirit over matter, of Creator over creation, [was] central to the new corpuscularian philosophy." I do not believe the lines should be so sharply drawn here. God for both Descartes and the corpuscularians was above nature; motion, not spirit per se, was primary for the corpuscularians. That God provided the initial impetus for motion and maintained an overseership was not something Descartes denied; the difference between the corpuscularians and Descartes was more in the choice of focus: for corpuscularians, a full explanation of natural phenomena had to include a discussion of final causes; Descartes' perspective was fixed on efficient causes.

42. Henry, "Occult Qualities," 344.

43. Ibid., 357, 336.

44. Clericuzio, "Redefinition," 583.

45. "Three Considerations about Subordinate Forms," in *Origin of Forms and Qualities, Works,* 3:127–28.

46. Thomas S. Hall, *Ideas of Life and Matter: Studies in the History of General Physiology, 600 B.C.–1900 A.D.,* 2 vols. (Chicago: University of Chicago Press, 1969), 1:19–20.

47. *Origin of Forms and Qualities, Works,* 3:136.

48. Dudley Shapere, "Plausibility and Justification in the Development of Science," *Journal of Philosophy* 63 (1966): 611–27.

49. *Origin of Forms and Qualities, Works,* 3:123.

50. Ibid., 3:127.

51. Ibid., 3:125–27, passim.

52. Hall, *Ideas of Life and Matter,* 1:284.

53. Roger French has argued that Sauvages's perspective on the body-machine is ultimately an "animistic" one ("Sickness and the Soul: Stahl, Hoffmann, and Sauvages on Pathology," in *The Medical Enlightenment of the Eighteenth Century,* ed. Andrew Cunningham and Roger French [Cambridge: Cambridge University Press, 1990], 106).

54. *Origin of Forms and Qualities, Works,* 3:124.

55. *Sceptical Chymist,* ibid., 1:500 and passim.

56. *Origin of Forms and Qualities,* ibid., 3:32, 68.

57. "A Physico-Chymical Essay containing an Experiment relating to Salt-Petre," in *Certain Physiological Essays,* ibid., 1:373.

58. See Clericuzio, "Redefinition," 583–87.

59. Ibid., 586, citing BP 2, fol. 141v.

60. Aristotle, for example, notes that once the principle of motion has been imparted to the parts of animals, "one thing follows on after another without interruption, just as it does in the 'miraculous' automatic puppets" (*Generation of Animals* 2.5.741b8).

61. This treatise, along with Descartes' *Treatise on Light* and another work, not extant, entitled *On the Soul,* were intended to make up a comprehensive tract

to be called *The World.* This work was never published, and it is thought that its deliberate suppression by Descartes was due to his concern over church censure, since this was the period in which Galileo was facing charges by the church for his espousal of Copernican ideas.

62. In his *Principles of Philosophy,* pt. 4, principle 203, Descartes explains that one is justified in making inferences of this type, noting that all knowledge man can have of nature is referable to the principles of geometry and mechanics and that understanding of the mechanical principles of perceived objects (either natural or contrived) will permit one to infer that the same mechanical principles apply at the subvisible level.

63. René Descartes, *Discourse on Method,* trans. Laurence J. Lafleur (New York: Bobbs-Merrill, 1956), 27.

64. Descartes maintained that the human embryo is formed from material nearly identical to that which composes the heavens. He closely related the development of the human organism around the central heart to the development of the heavenly bodies around a central sun. For more information on this see Richard B. Carter, *Descartes' Medical Philosophy: The Organic Solution to the Mind-Body Problem* (Baltimore: Johns Hopkins University Press, 1983), 191–212.

65. *Free Inquiry into the Vulgarly Received Notion of Nature, Works,* 5:232.

66. Boyle deals extensively with this subject in his *Essays of the Strange Subtilty, great Efficacy, determinate Nature of Effluviums* and "Of the Porousness of Animal Bodies," published in 1673 and 1684, respectively.

67. *Free Inquiry, Works,* 5:235.

68. "Meditation I: Upon the First Invasion of the Disease," in *Occasional Reflections,* ibid., 2:366–67.

69. Although this view provides some parameters for the individual to operate on his own behalf, I do not hold that Boyle here is attempting to find an avenue for the expression of free will. Boyle's argument, taken in context, is still focused on the power of God and the complexity of the design of nature. He is trying to make the point that it is inadequate to look upon the human body as an automaton, for the human body is a far more sophisticated mechanism than is suggested by that term (*Free Inquiry,* ibid., 5:236). For a person to use reason to attempt to avoid physical danger does not compromise the notion of predestination; in "reacting," man could still be playing out a predetermined role, however unaware he might be of doing so.

70. Ibid.

71. *The Christian Virtuoso. The Second Part, Works,* 6:754.

72. Christoph Meinel, "Empirical Support for the Corpuscular Theory in the Seventeenth Century," in *Theory and Experiment: Recent Insights and New Perspectives on Their Relation,* ed. Diderik Batens and Jean Paul (Dordrecht: Reidel, 1988), 89.

Chapter 3 The Augmentation of Medical Knowledge

1. See Frank, *Harvey and Oxford.*

2. Harvey worked at Oxford in 1645–46, in close collaboration with

Nathaniel Highmore, Charles Scarburgh, George and Ralph Bathurst, Walter Charleton, and the young Thomas Willis. These men, all of whom later became associates of Boyle's, utilized many of Harvey's methods in their own investigations. For a description of Harvey's work at Oxford see ibid., 21–30.

3. *Usefulness of Experimental Natural Philosophy, Works,* 2:13–14.

4. *Appendix to the Second Part of the Christian Virtuoso,* ibid., 6:731.

5. *Usefulness of Experimental Natural Philosophy,* ibid., 2:73.

6. Ibid., 2:73–75.

7. See comments by Birch, "Life of Boyle," ibid., 1:lviii; and Turnbull, "Samuel Hartlib's Influence," 124.

8. *Usefulness of Experimental Natural Philosophy,* pt. 2, essay 1, *Works,* 2:67.

9. Ibid., 2:68–69.

10. Ibid., 2:67.

11. For an analysis of Boyle's views on the moral justification for animal experimentation and how he reconciled this with an ethical obligation toward humane treatment of animals see Malcolm R. Oster, "The 'Beaume of Diuinity': Animal Suffering in the Early Thought of Robert Boyle," *British Journal for the History of Science* 22 (1989): 151–79.

12. For further discussion of Harvey's views and how they differed from Galen's see Frank, *Harvey and Oxford,* 2–16.

13. Ibid., 20.

14. *New Experiments . . . Touching the Spring of the Air, Works,* 1:99–113. The information contained in the next several paragraphs is from this same source, 1:100–108.

15. Some of these were based on experiments in his own vacuum receiver; some were based on experiments of others. He cites, for example, the observation that "fishes soon die in ponds and glasses quite filled with water; if the one be so frozen over, and the other so closely stopped, that the fishes cannot enjoy the benefit of the air." Boyle adds his own suggestion that since, as experimental evidence has shown, there are "many little parcels of interspersed air" within water, fish may utilize this air to live (ibid., 1:109).

16. Ibid., 1:113.

17. On this see Frank, *Harvey and Oxford;* and Henry Guerlac, "John Mayow and the Aerial Niter: Studies in the Chemistry of John Mayow, I," *Actes du Septième Congrès International d'Histoire des Sciences* (Jerusalem, 1953), 332–39, and "Studies in the Chemistry of John Mayow: II. The Poet's Nitre," *Isis* 45 (1954): 243–55. Guerlac maintains that the idea that niter possesses a vital power originated with the attempts to explain the meteorological phenomena of lightning and thunder by analogy with the explosion of gunpowder (which contains niter as an essential ingredient).

18. Both Seton and Sendivogius wrote of a "dew" of life that vitalized plants (Frank, *Harvey and Oxford,* 119). These notions were an extension of the larger chemical world view of Paracelsus (see Debus, *Chemical Philosophy,* 1:87–88).

19. Digby held that saltpeter fertilized because it "attracteth a like Salt that Foecundateth the Aire" (see Frank, *Harvey and Oxford,* 126–27).

Notes to Pages 79–86

20. See the entry for 17 June 1667 in Thomas Birch, *History of the Royal Society*, 4 vols. (London, 1757), 2:184.

21. Lower's research on this subject was published as *Tractatus de corde item de motu et colore sanguinis et chyli in eum transitu* (London, 1669).

22. Willis' comments are found in part 1 of his *Affectionum quae dicituntur hystericae et hypocondriacae . . . cui accesserunt exercitationes medico-physicae duae* (London, 1670).

23. "A Physico-Chymical Essay . . . relating to Salt-Petre," *Works*, 1:371–72.

24. "New Pneumatical Experiments about Respiration: A Continuation," title 15, ibid., 3:382–83. What Boyle did not realize, of course, was that carbon dioxide had replaced oxygen in his receiver in the same volume.

25. See, e.g., *New Experiments . . . Touching the Spring of the Air*, ibid., 1:11; "An Experimental Discourse of some Unheeded Causes of the Insalubrity and Salubrity of the Air," ibid., 5:44; and elsewhere.

26. *New Experiments touching the Relation betwixt Flame and Air*, title 1, ibid., 3:570.

27. Boyle's "New Pneumatical Experiments about Respiration," title 5, "Experiments on the question of whether air is usually harbored and concealed in the pores of water," discusses this issue (ibid., 3:361–63).

28. *New Experiments touching the Relation betwixt Flame and Air*, experiment 5, ibid., 3:577.

29. Frank, *Harvey and Oxford*, 253.

30. *New Experiments about the Relation between Air and the Flamma Vitalis of Animals*, *Works*, 3:587–88.

31. *New Experiments . . . Touching the Spring of the Air*, ibid., 1:99.

32. *Suspicions about some Hidden Qualities of the Air*, ibid., 4:85.

33. Ibid., 4:90.

34. Ibid.

35. Ibid., 4:91.

36. Douglas McKie, "Fire and the Flamma Vitalis: Boyle, Hooke, and Mayow," in *Science, Medicine, and History: Essays in Honour of Charles Singer*, ed. E. A. Underwood, 2 vols. (London: Oxford University Press, 1953), 1:485.

37. Westfall, in fact, sees Mayow's interpretation as a good example of the joining of a Hermetic concept of active principles with a mechanistic interpretation and observes that "the mere translation of the nitroaerial spirit into mechanistic language clearly changed very little in the concept itself" (Richard S. Westfall, "Newton and the Hermetic Tradition," in *Science, Medicine, and Society in the Renaissance: Essays to Honour Walter Pagel*, ed. Allen G. Debus, 2 vols. [New York: Science History Publications, 1972], 2:188).

38. *History of the Air*, *Works*, 5:627.

39. Ibid., 5:628.

40. Ibid., 5:627.

41. *Usefulness of Experimental Natural Philosophy*, ibid., 2:80. Many of the chemists, of course, wished to abandon Galenic theory altogether. Galen's equilibrium model involved the notion that disease was ultimately an expression of

humoral imbalance, which the physician rectified by purging excess humors and fortifying depleted ones. This was inconsistent with iatrochemical theories based on disease as a specific entity that had to be expunged or neutralized. The information contained in the next several paragraphs is from this same source, 2:80–152.

42. "The History of Fluidity and Firmness. The First Part, of Fluidity," in *Certain Physiological Essays,* ibid., 1:381.

43. *Usefulness of Experimental Natural Philosophy,* ibid., 2:127. This view of a powerful solvent in the stomach was one Boyle shared with his Paracelsian colleagues.

44. Ibid., 2:127.

45. Ibid., 2:79, 72.

46. As late as 1683 we find Boyle still referring to the existence of gastric acid as an idea ascribed to by "Helmont and his disciples, [and] a great part of the modern chymists, and physicians too" (*The Natural History of Human Blood,* ibid., 4:622). If Boyle had acquired evidence of his own by this time, he certainly would have noted it.

47. Recorded in Hartlib's *Ephemerides* for 1658, quoted in Turnbull, "Samuel Hartlib's Influence," 115.

48. A discussion of Wren's transfusion experiments is provided in Dorothy Stimson, *Scientists and Amateurs: A History of the Royal Society* (New York: Henry Schuman, 1948), 84.

49. *Philosophical Transactions of the Royal Society of London,* no. 20, p. 353, for Monday, 17 December 1666, *Works,* 3:149–51.

50. Ibid., no. 22, p. 385, for Monday, 11 February 1666, *Works,* 3:152–53.

51. Frank, *Harvey and Oxford,* 185.

52. B.L. M–P, no. 10, quoted in Howard B. Adelmann, *Marcello Malpighi and the Evolution of Embryology,* 5 vols. (Ithaca: Cornell University Press, 1966), 1:268. Malpighi was first to describe the red blood corpuscles (the "red atometti") in his treatise *De polypo cordis* (1666), but he never recognized the significance of his discovery. We have no comments from Boyle on this subject.

53. *Natural History of Human Blood, Works,* 4:619, 620.

54. *Of the Reconcileableness of Specific Medicines to the Corpuscular Philosophy,* ibid., 5:97.

Chapter 4 The Human Body and the Environment

1. Clarence J. Glacken, *Traces on the Rhodian Shore: Nature and Culture in Western Thought from Ancient Times to the End of the Eighteenth Century* (Berkeley and Los Angeles: University of California Press, 1973), 462. Glacken notes that even though Europeans in the Middle Ages knew that means of altering nature existed (e.g., through clearing trees, draining swamps, etc.), a "bolder synthesis" occurred in the seventeenth and eighteenth centuries by which the potential for humans to effect their environment was extolled.

2. Ibid., 358, 432, and passim.

3. For a fuller discussion see Frederick Sargent, *Hippocratic Heritage: A History of Ideas about Weather and Human Health* (New York: Pergamon, 1982), 64.

4. James C. Riley, *The Eighteenth Century Campaign to Avoid Disease* (New York: Macmillan, 1987), ix.

5. Ibid., 9–51.

6. Ibid., xii.

7. *Origin of Forms and Qualities, Works,* 3:20.

8. *Free Inquiry,* ibid., 5:177.

9. Ibid., 5:179.

10. *Origin of Forms and Qualities,* ibid., 3:26.

11. *A Disquisition about the Final Causes of Natural Things,* ibid., 5:440.

12. *Usefulness of Experimental Natural Philosophy,* ibid., 2:76. Boyle's complaint with the Paracelsians was that they saw the macrocosm and the microcosm as made up of identical entities, such that every part of the macrocosm had its physical or spiritual counterpart within the human body. Boyle's schema, on the other hand, postulated only an identity of *operations* between the two realms, not spiritual linkages.

13. See *Free Inquiry,* ibid., 5:218–40.

14. Ibid., 5:221.

15. Whether to define disease as physiological or ontological was hotly debated in the seventeenth century. Many contemporary writers have addressed this subject; see esp. Owsei Temkin, "The Scientific Approach to Disease: Specific Entities and Individual Sickness," *The Double Face of Janus* (Baltimore: Johns Hopkins University Press, 1977), 441-55, and Peter Niebyl, "Sennert, Van Helmont, and Medical Ontology," *Bulletin of the History of Medicine* 45 (1971): 115–37.

16. Niebyl, "Sennert, Van Helmont, and Medical Ontology," 123. Niebyl explains that a physiological interpretation of disease need not automatically imply a physiological interpretation of disease causation.

17. See *Free Inquiry, Works,* 5:233.

18. Boyle insisted that even imagined factors had physical sources, which was necessary if he were to maintain his position that all diseases, or more properly, disorders, had physical causes. In *Appendix to the First Part of the Christian Virtuoso,* he states: "That faculty, which is called fantasy or imagination, is a corporeal faculty, and exercised but about such things as were introduced into the mind by the senses or are compounded of such images, or derived from them" (ibid., 6:685).

19. Boyle, like other mechanical philosophers, had great difficulty explaining how mind acted on body. He chose not to become involved with this subject in his writings, preferring simply to postulate this separate "supra- mechanical" category of operations. His justification for utilizing such a category was based on an argument from design:

> The consideration of the nature and properties of the unmatched union of the body and mind of man has, I confess, sometime invited and inclined me to venture upon making a distinction, that appears not to have yet occurred to philosophers, or divines. For instead of dividing the operations of God, here below, into two sorts only, natural and supernatural; I think we may take in a third sort, and divide the same operations into supernatural, natural, in a stricter sense, that is mechanical, and natural in a larger sense, which I call supra-mechanical. For whereas all the phaenomena of the world, as it is an aggregate, or system of mere bodies, are performed by matter, and local motion, according to mechanical laws; the operations of the human mind, and its organical body upon one another, are not to be accounted for by mere matter, and its mechanical powers. . . . So that these operations, that belong to a man as he is so, though in some sense they are not supernatural, because the order of things being once established by the most wise and powerful author of them, they are produced according to the course of nature; yet they may be stiled supra-mechanical, because they cannot be mechanically explicated or produced, nor can they be proved to flow from natural causes, if these are considered, as but corporeal ones. (*The Christian Virtuoso. The Second Part,* ibid., 6:754)

20. The history of the concept of effluvia is provided by Gordon K. Chalmers in "Effluvia, the History of a Metaphor," *Modern Language Association of America Publications* 52 (1937): 1031–50; "Three Terms of the Corpuscularian Philosophy," *Modern Philology* 33 (1936): 243-60; and "The Lodestone and the Understanding of Matter in Seventeenth Century England," *Philosophy of Science* 4 (1937): 75–95.

21. *Essays of the . . . determinate Nature of Effluviums, Works,* 3:689.

22. Boyle provides several examples to show that effluvia could retain the properties characteristic of the emitting body: water vapor, for instance, condenses back into water; and quicksilver, once distilled, could condense back into running mercury. It was crucial to Boyle's argument of the effects of effluvia on bodies to assume that they remained chemically identical to the emitting body, even though their physical form was different (see ibid., 3:691).

23. Boyle did not deny that celestial objects could emit effluvia, since to do so would have been logically inconsistent with his postulate that all bodies could emit effluvia. However, because of the great distances involved, he maintained that celestial effluvia would have far less effect on terrestrial bodies than would effluvia emanating from terrestrial objects (see "Insalubrity and Salubrity of the Air," ibid., 5:51).

24. *Essays of the . . . determinate Nature of Effluviums,* ibid., 3:678.

25. Ibid., 3:677–78.

26. "Insalubrity and Salubrity of the Air," ibid., 5:45.

27. *History of the Air,* ibid., 5:613–14.

28. See *New Experiments . . . Touching the Spring of the Air,* experiment 29, ibid., 1:66.

29. "Insalubrity and Salubrity of the Air," ibid., 5:44.

30. *Suspicions about some Hidden Qualities of the Air,* ibid., 4:86; *History of the Air,* ibid., 5:713.

31. *Origin and Virtues of Gems,* ibid., 3:544.

32. *History of Cold,* ibid., 2:587.

33. "Of the Temperature of the Subterraneal Regions," ibid., 3:336.

34. Aristotle's comments are found in his *Meteorologica* 3.6.378a.

35. See Debus, *Chemical Philosophy,* 1:89.

36. See Hartlib to Boyle, 8 May 1654, which refers to Glauber (*Works,* 6:86), and Boyle's descriptions of Glauber's furnaces in *Usefulness of Experimental Natural Philosophy* (ibid., 2:139).

37. Johann Rudolph Glauber, *Of the Nature of Salts* (1658), cited in Debus, *Chemical Philosophy,* 2:433.

38. *Cosmical Suspicions, Works,* 3:318–19.

39. *Origin and Virtues of Gems,* ibid., 3:558.

40. Boyle makes note of this point frequently. See, e.g., his comments in *Suspicions about some Hidden Qualities of the Air,* ibid., 4:94.

41. "Of the Porousness of Animal Bodies," ibid., 4:770.

42. This, for Boyle, was an important consideration in drug therapy:

> It is possible for the subtil effluvia of several bodies to get through the pores of the skin; and when they have once got admittance, so much as into the smaller vessels, it is easy to conceive, how these may carry them into the greater, and consequently into the mass of blood, by whose circulation they may be readily conveyed to all parts of the body, and among them to the seat of the disease: and perhaps (to add that upon the bye), the efficacy of these corpuscles, that, if I may so speak, get in at the key-hole, not at the door, may be the more considerable, because they get presently into the mass of blood, without passing through those digestions in the stomach and other parts, which oftentimes much weaken the virtue of medicines taken in at the mouth before they arrive at the blood. (*Reconcileableness of Specific Medicines,* ibid., 5:87)

43. *Natural History of Human Blood,* ibid., 4:641.

44. *Cosmical Suspicions,* ibid., 3:311. By the seventeenth century, physicians had become acquainted with a variety of "new diseases" not mentioned by the ancient medical authors, two of the most obvious examples being syphilis and rickets.

45. "Insalubrity and Salubrity of the Air," ibid., 5:50.

46. "The Plague of London from the Hand of God," BP 14, item 2, fols. 28r–42v.

47. "Insalubrity and Salubrity of the Air," *Works,* 5:58. The information contained in the next several paragraphs is from this same source, 5:46–61.

Notes to Pages 108–113

48. More, *Life and Works of Boyle,* 117.

49. Samuel Colepresse to Boyle, 1 February 1666/67, *Works,* 6:548–52.

50. Debus, *Chemical Philosophy,* 1:15.

51. For example, as Debus relates, "By 1571 Leonard Thurneisser was using quantitative methods, solubility tests, crystallographic evidence, and some flame tests in an attempt to determine the active substances in spa waters" (ibid., 1:110–11). At the end of the sixteenth century, Libavius employed these methods along with the oak gall test. Debus notes, "One can trace a growing interest in analytical color tests in the work of Paracelsians throughout the early years of the seventeenth century" (1:112).

52. Ibid.

53. Boyle includes many more specific areas of investigation than are noted here (see *Short Memoirs for the Natural Experimental History of Mineral Waters,* sec. 6, *Works,* 4:818-20).

54. The inspiration for this work was, of course, Hippocrates' treatise *Airs, Waters, and Places,* one of his most lasting and most influential works.

55. Willis states: "Following the example of Hippocrates, we first consider the foregoing constitution of the Year; its intemperance and excess of qualities. For Epidemical Diseases, commonly excited among the people, there will be a Common Cause, such as is to be assigned to the habit of the Year, whence a disposition of our Blood is contracted whereby many people are affected equally" (*On Feavers,* quoted in Donald G. Bates, "Thomas Willis and the Epidemic Fever of 1661: A Commentary," *Bulletin of the History of Medicine* 39 [1965]: 403).

56. Isbrand van Diemerbroeck, *A Treatise concerning the Pestilence,* trans. Thomas Stanton (London, 1722), preface and chap. 1. For Boyle's comments concerning this treatise see "Insalubrity and Salubrity of the Air," *Works,* 5:63.

57. *History of the Air,* ibid., 5:640. Note that Boyle does not suggest any direct occult influences of celestial bodies upon the human body. The link is between planetary positions and weather conditions, conditions that could, in turn, give rise to additional specific factors causing illness. "It cannot be denied," Boyle writes, "but all the affections and dispositions of moisture, heat, cold, drought, the course of all winds, showers, thundering, or whatsoever else is used by nature, to produce . . . universal effects of rarefaction and condensation, do in great measure, if not wholly, depend upon, and are altogether regulated by, the course, motion, position, situations or aspects, of the superior and celestial bodies or planets" (ibid.).

58. "Two Essays concerning the Unsuccessfulness of Experiments: First Essay—Of the Unsuccessfulness of Experiments," ibid., 1:327.

59. *Of Men's Great Ignorance of the Uses of Natural Things,* ibid., 3:473.

60. *Essays of the . . . determinate Nature of Effluviums,* ibid., 3:698.

61. *Usefulness of Experimental Natural Philosophy,* ibid., 2:179.

62. *Essays of the . . . determinate Nature of Effluviums,* ibid., 3:699.

63. "A New Experiment Concerning an Effect of the Varying Weight of the Atmosphere upon Some Bodies in the Water; suggesting a Conjecture, that the very Alterations of the Air, in point of Weight, may have Considerable Opera-

tions, even upon Men's Sickness or Health," *Philosophical Transactions of the Royal Society of London,* 24 February 1672/73, ibid., 3:656.

64. *History of the Air,* ibid., 5:692.

65. "A New Experiment and other Instances of the Efficacy of the Air's Moisture," *Tracts Consisting of Observations about the saltness of the sea,* ibid., 3:798–99.

66. *History of the Air,* ibid., 5:642.

67. Ibid., 5:655–83.

68. See James H. Cassedy, "Medicine and the Rise of Statistics," in Debus, *Medicine in Seventeenth Century England,* 283–312. As Cassedy notes regarding Locke's ambitious goals of meteorological data gathering, "While Locke's global inquiry did not yield much in the way of data, it was not an outlandish project; it was only premature" (304).

Chapter 5 The Restoration of Health

1. *Usefulness of Experimental Natural Philosophy, Works,* 2:161.

2. Ibid., 2:181.

3. *Reconcileableness of Specific Medicines,* ibid., 5:84 (emphasis added).

4. *Free Inquiry,* ibid., 5:231. The information contained in the next several paragraphs is from this same source, 5:211–37.

5. *Reconcileableness of Specific Medicines, Works,* 5:84–85.

6. According to Boyle, "Specifics, where they can be had, are wont to be free from any immoderate manifest quality, and for the most part . . . work more benignly, as well as more effectually, *caeteris paribus,* than other medicines" (ibid., 5:75).

7. Ibid., 5:86.

8. See Boyle's comments in *Natural History of Human Blood,* ibid., 4:641.

9. *Usefulness of Experimental Natural Philosophy,* ibid., 2:191–92.

10. Comments on Greatrakes provided here are largely drawn from Barbara Beigun Kaplan, "Greatrakes the Stroker: The Interpretations of His Contemporaries," *Isis* 73 (1982): 178–85.

11. Boyle held that passions manifested themselves in terms of physical corpuscular movements by "supra-mechanical" means.

12. This episode involving Boyle's participation in the curing performance is described by the physician James Faireclough in a letter to Sir William Smith, 5 May 1666. The letter is included in [Valentine Greatraks,] *A Brief Account of Mr. Valentine Greatraks, and Divers of the Strange Cases by Him Lately Performed* (London, 1666), 71. Boyle never considered that the patient's "cure" might have been due to the power of suggestion.

13. The list is in BL, 3, vol. 33. It was appended to a letter from Boyle to Henry Stubbe dated 9 March 1665/66. The printed version of this letter (*Works,* 1:lxxv–lxxxv) does not contain the list of queries; however, Maddison has reproduced it in his biography of Boyle (Maddison, *Life,* 124–26).

14. Oldenburg wrote Boyle in March 1666, "Greatrix does certainly some cures by his frictions, insinuating (perhaps) some salubrious steams or spirits of

his own into sickly people's bodies" (Oldenburg to Boyle, 13 March 1666, *Works,* 6:221).

15. *Usefulness of Experimental Natural Philosophy,* ibid., 2:128.

16. For example, an entry in one of Boyle's commonplace books reads: "There are divers Mineral Preparations, wherein a Drug is so . . . combined and perhaps compounded with others, or so artificially disguis'd by Preparations, that tis hard to discover it to be either the Principal Ingredient, or perhaps any Ingredient at all, by Taste, Smell, or the Common Ways of Investigating what a propos'd Medicine is made of. Now in such cases as these Reduction may be of considerable use; for a sagacious and skilfull Artist may find Wayes to pull off the visors from Minerals that would remain perpetually disguis'd to the generality of Naturalists and Physicians" (RS MS. 199, fol. 19r).

17. Boyle argued, "[The naturalist] may, by his several ways of trial, and by his chymical preparations discover, that divers bodies, especially of a mineral nature that are as yet not at all imployed by physicians, at least internally, may be brought into use by them; and that others, that are naturally so dangerous, as to be used but in very few, and for the most part extreme cases, may with safety be more freely employed" (*Usefulness of Experimental Natural Philosophy, Works,* 2:119–20).

18. Ibid., 2:117.

19. RS MS. 199, fol. 44v.

20. *Usefulness of Experimental Natural Philosophy, Works,* 2:127.

21. "An Appendix to the First Section of the Second Part," *Usefulness of Experimental Natural Philosophy,* ibid., 2:241 (emphasis added).

22. "Advantages of the Use of Simple Medicines," ibid., 5:116.

23. Ibid., 5:109.

24. Ibid., 5:124.

25. Boas, *Robert Boyle and Seventeenth-Century Chemistry,* 30. 33. The essay on poisons was written at about the same time as part 1 of *Usefulness of Experimental Natural Philosophy,* probably in the early 1650s.

26. Debus, *Chemical Philosophy,* 1:541–42.

27. *Usefulness of Experimental Natural Philosophy, Works,* 2:28.

28. "Insalubrity and Salubrity of the Air," ibid., 5:63. As noted earlier, Boyle believed orpiment (arsenic trisulfide) to be a possible cause of plague.

29. "Essay of Turning Poisons into Medicines," RS MS. 1.

30. *Medicina Hydrostatica, Works,* 5:453–507.

31. Sanctorio Sanctorius (1551–1636) was a pioneer in physiology (particularly the physiology of metabolism), introducing exact methods of measurement, weighing, and pulse counting, for which he developed new instruments, such as the clinical thermometer and the pulse clock. The highly innovative treatise of Sanctorius to which Boyle refers was published in 1614 and contains a description of the Paduan professor's famous attempt to measure "insensible perspiration" by weighing himself in a balance chair. Boyle, no doubt, chose a parallel title for his own treatise to indicate his belief that he was breaking new ground in a similar fashion.

32. Ibid., 5:454.

Chapter 6 Boyle's Medical Thought in Its Contemporary Context

1. See Marie Boas Hall, "Boyle's Method of Work: Promoting His Corpuscular Philosophy," *Notes and Records of the Royal Society of London* 41 (1987): 111. Hall points out that at any given time, Boyle had many drafts and fragments of treatises on hand, and he kept these in his possession for years without publishing them. Despite his plan to write comprehensive works both on the corpuscular view of nature and on a system of chemistry, he often preferred to scavenge ideas and experiments from drafts of earlier unpublished treatises for placement in others. Frequently, his papers were lost due to carelessness.

2. Boss, "The 'Methodus Medendi' as an Index of Change," 30–32. Boss points out that the logical structure of the inquiry into disease, as well as the cardiovascular physiology embedded in Galenic *methodus medendi,* was under attack at this time.

3. RS MS. 199, fol. 120r. Michael Hunter identifies these as passages of a suppressed work "Considerations & Doubts Touching the Vulgar Method of Physick."

4. Ibid., fol. 117v.

5. It is interesting to conjecture how much Boyle's intense opposition to excessively violent evacuations may have stemmed from the early incident in his childhood when at school he was mistakenly given a strong purgative meant for another patient and became seriously ill as a result.

6. Ibid., fol. 115v–115r.

7. *Usefulness of Experimental Natural Philosophy, Works,* 2:199.

8. Ibid., 2:185–86.

9. *Certain Physiological Essays,* ibid., 1:308 (emphasis added).

10. Ibid., 1:309–10.

11. *Essays of the . . . determinate Nature of Effluviums,* ibid., 3:661.

12. On Sennert see Andrew G. Van Melsen, *From Atomos to Atom* (New York: Harper Torchbooks, 1960), 81–89; on Sennert and Boyle's opinion of him see Marie Boas [Hall], "The Establishment of the Mechanical Philosophy," *Osiris* 10 (1952): 438–39; and on Digby see Robert Kargon, *Atomism in England from Hariot to Newton* (Oxford: Clarendon Press, 1966), 72–73, and Lester King, *The Road to Medical Enlightenment* (New York: Science History Publications, 1970), 140–45.

13. See the discussion in chapter 2.

14. Shapin and Schaffer have delineated the social dimensions of the process of generating and validating knowledge (*Leviathan and the Air-Pump,* 23–79 and passim).

15. Harold J. Cook, "Physicians and the New Philosophy: Henry Stubbe and the Virtuosi-Physicians," in French and Wear, *Medical Revolution of the Seventeenth Century,* 248.

16. Roy Porter, "The Early Royal Society and the Spread of Medical Knowledge," in ibid., 280.

17. R. Palmer, "Life of the Most Eminent Dr. Baldwin Hamey" (1733), manuscript at Royal College of Physicians, quoted in Maddison, *Life,* 137.

18. Michael Hunter suggests that such tentativeness of expression, though characteristic of his *published* works, was not necessarily characteristic of Boyle's *manuscript* writings (unpublished paper).

19. Mandelbaum, *Philosophy, Science, and Sense Perception,* 63.

20. Shapin and Schaffer, *Leviathan and the Air-Pump,* chap. 4.

21. Ibid., 140. As Shapin and Schaffer point out, Hobbes consistently treated hypotheses derived from experiments as "statements about real causes" (111).

22. For a more detailed discussion see ibid., 170–207. The quotation is from p. 176.

23. Kenneth D. Keele, "The Sydenham-Boyle Theory of Morbific Particles," *Medical History* 18 (1974): 240, 247.

24. Cunningham, "Thomas Sydenham," 180.

25. John Locke to Thomas Molyneux, 20 January 1692/93, quoted in Kenneth Dewhurst, *Dr. Thomas Sydenham (1624–1689): His Life and Writings* (Berkeley: University of California Press, 1966), 179.

26. *Usefulness of Experimental Natural Philosophy, Works,* 2:185.

27. Thomas Sydenham, *The Works of Thomas Sydenham, M.D.,* trans. and ed. R. G. Latham, 2 vols. (London: Sydenham Society, 1848–50), 2:83–84, quoted in David E. Wolfe, "Sydenham and Locke on the Limits of Anatomy," *Bulletin of the History of Medicine* 35 (1961): 202. Sydenham's focus is on how disease "evolves," not what causes it.

28. For this reason, Sydenham's method was far more palatable than Boyle's for those who wished to maintain themselves as professionals separate from the general community.

29. Patrick Romanell, *John Locke and Medicine: A New Key to Locke* (Buffalo, N.Y.: Prometheus Books, 1984), 113. The information in the next several paragraphs is from this same source, 106–12.

30. Ibid., 114, quoting Locke's "Anatomia" manuscript, Public Records Office, London, 30/24/47/No. 2, fol. 60.

31. Quoted in ibid., 114.

32. RS MS 186, fols. 19r–20r.

Chapter 7 Boyle's Legacy

1. Cook, "Physicians and the New Philosophy," 268.

2. See Cook, *Decline,* esp. chap. 4.

3. *Usefulness of Experimental Natural Philosophy, Works,* 2:4.

4. According to John Maddison, Boyle's biographer, Boyle did some of this work at Gresham College in 1661 and 1662 (Maddison, *Life,* 102, 110).

5. H. Chamberlen to Boyle, 17 January 1665/66, BL, vol. 2, nos. 5, 7, and 8, cited in Maddison, *Life,* 122–23. Maddison suggests that Hugh Chamberlen was probably the son of Peter Chamberlen.

6. "Some Uncommon Observations about Vitiated Sight," appended to *Disquisition about the Final Causes of Things,* in *Works,* 5:445. In this short appendix Boyle describes and comments upon the examinations he has made of a number of individuals suffering from distinctive eye disorders. It is possible that Boyle's

particular interest in eye disorders was due to his own lifelong vision problems.

7. Maddison, *Life,* 122. Daubeny Turberville (1612–96) was an Oxford-educated oculist who practiced in Salisbury and in London. Boyle had referred Pepys to Turberville for eye treatment (Samuel Pepys, *The Diary of Samuel Pepys,* ed. Robert Latham and William Matthews, 11 vols. [London: G. Bell, 1970–83], entry for 22 June 1668).

8. Michael Hunter, *The Royal Society and Its Fellows: 1660–1700: The Morphology of an Early Scientific Institution,* British Society for the History of Science Monograph, 4 (London, 1982), 24.

9. See Cook, *Decline,* 165.

10. A. Rupert Hall, "Medicine and the Royal Society," in Debus, *Medicine in Seventeenth Century England,* 424.

11. On Merrett's position and the debate within the Royal College of Physicians in general concerning the value of the new philosophy to medicine see Cook, "Physicians and the New Philosophy," 256.

12. In a work entitled *The Character of a Compleat Physician, or Naturalist,* published in London in 1680, Merrett urged physicians to know nature and to acquire knowledge of the operations of drugs. Cook notes that this work was attributed to Merrett by Anthony Wood in *Athenae Oxoniensis* (London, 1692), vol. 6, cols. 430–32 (see Cook, *Decline,* 167–68).

13. Hamey's strong opposition to the Royal Society may have been personal as well as professional, since Hamey was ousted as an officer of the Royal College of Physicians in 1667, when a group of younger men, including Merrett, who were more sympathetic to the new science were elected to the executive positions.

14. Cook, *Decline,* 179.

15. Ibid., 181.

16. A. R. Hall, "Medicine and the Royal Society," 430, citing *Usefulness of Experimental Natural Philosophy,* pt. 2, essay 5, *Works,* 2:170.

17. Ibid., 430–31.

18. *Reconcileableness of Specific Medicines, Works,* 5:74.

19. Lester King, *The Growth of Medical Thought* (Chicago: University of Chicago Press, 1963), 159–74.

20. Friedrich Hoffmann, *Fundamenta Medicinae,* translated with an introduction by Lester S. King (New York: Neale Watson, 1971), 2.

21. King, *Growth of Medical Thought,* 163–64, translating Hoffmann, *Medicina rationalis systematica,* 2d ed., 8 vols in 4 (Halle, 1729–39), 1:19. The Latin reads: "Attenta observatione discimus, motum omnium mutationum in corporeis causam esse, atque motu quoque vitae ac sanitatis fundamentum contineri, ipsas morborum causas vix alio modo, quam motu, in corporis nostri solidas & fluidas partes agere, neque medicamenta aliter, quam motu, operationes exserere. Qua de causa in explanadis medicis rebus inque remediorum viribus explicandis, ad motum principaliter, deinde ad mobile, sive dispositionem corporum ipsasque vias, respiciendum esse existimamus."

22. Ibid., 175, translating Hoffmann, *Medicina rationalis systematica,* 1:75.

23. See French, "Sickness and the Soul," 92.

Notes to Pages 156–162

24. King, *Growth of Medical Thought,* 165–66.

25. Andrew Cunningham, "Medicine to Calm the Mind: Boerhaave's Medical System, and Why It Was Adopted in Edinburgh," in Cunningham and French, *Medical Enlightenment of the Eighteenth Century,* 48, 55. Cunningham suggests that Boyle's own irenicism served as a model for Boerhaave.

26. Hermann Boerhaave, *A New Method of Chemistry,* trans. Peter Shaw and E. Chambers (London, 1727), 46–47, quoted in Maddison, *Life,* 193.

27. Riley, *Eighteenth Century Campaign to Avoid Disease,* 12–13.

28. Ibid., 28.

29. Ibid., 9.

30. An interesting account of this attitude and its societal dimensions is given in Roy Porter, "Lay Medical Knowledge in the Eighteenth Century: The Evidence of *The Gentlemen's Magazine,*" *Medical History* 29 (1958): 138–68.

31. Peter Shaw, *An enquiry into the contents, virtues and uses of the Scarborough Spaw waters, with the method of examining any other mineral water* (London, 1734), 7. For a good summary of eighteenth-century work on mineral waters see Noel G. Coley, "Physicians and the Chemical Analysis of Mineral Waters in Eighteenth-Century England," *Medical History* 26 (1982): 123–44.

32. Marina Benjamin, "Medicine, Morality, and the Politics of Berkeley's Tar-Water," in Cunningham and French, *Medical Enlightenment of the Eighteenth Century,* 183.

33. See Simon Schaffer, "Measuring Virtue: Eudiometry, Enlightenment, and Pneumatic Medicine," in ibid., 281–318.

34. On this process see ibid., 285–87; and J. R. Partington, *A Short History of Chemistry,* 3d ed. (New York: Harper Torchbooks, 1960), 113–15.

35. Priestley's test had some major flaws, including his equation of "respirability" with "goodness" and the difficulty of obtaining regular results unless care was taken to perform the test under standard conditions of temperature and pressure. This latter problem caused Priestley to proclaim that the "virtue" of the air differed significantly in places where there was in fact little difference at all (see Partington, *Short History of Chemistry,* 115).

36. Schaffer, "Measuring Virtue," esp. 292–318.

37. Cook, "Physicians and the New Philosophy," 247 (emphasis added).

38. See chap. 6.

39. Erwin H. Ackerknecht, *A Short History of Medicine,* rev. ed. (Baltimore: Johns Hopkins University Press, 1982), 129–30.

40. See N. D. Jewson, "Medical Knowledge and the Patronage System in Eighteenth-Century England," *Sociology* 8 (1974): 369–85, and "The Disappearance of the Sick Man from Medical Cosmology, 1770–1870," ibid. 10 (1976): 225–40.

41. Malcolm Nicolson, "The Metastatic Theory of Pathogenesis and the Professional Interests of the Eighteenth-Century Physician," *Medical History* 32 (1988): 277–300.

42. Anita Guerrini, "Newtonian Matter Theory, Chemistry, and Medicine, 1690–1713" (Ph.D. diss., Indiana University, 1983); idem, "Isaac Newton, George

Cheyne, and the *Principia Medicinae*," in French and Wear, *Medical Revolution of the Seventeenth Century*, 222–45.

43. Guerrini, "Newtonian Matter Theory," 135–36.

44. Steven Shapin, "Social Uses of Science," in *The Ferment of Knowledge: Studies in the Historiography of Eighteenth Century Science*, ed, G. S. Rousseau and Roy Porter (Cambridge: Cambridge University Press, 1980), 97, citing Frank Manuel, *A Portrait of Isaac Newton* (Cambridge: Harvard University Press, 1968).

45. Boyle had discussed this view of matter in his *Sceptical Chymist*. Basically it involved the idea that matter was made up of increasingly complex conglomerations of primary particles, differing in number and arrangement. Since the primary particles were identical, this meant that transmutation was possible.

46. See Guerrini, "Newtonian Matter Theory."

47. Ibid., 208–9.

48. Clericuzio, "Redefinition," 561.

49. Gottfried Wilhelm Leibniz to Christian Huygens, 29 December 1691, in *Oeuvres complétes de Christiaan Huygens, publiées par la Société Hollandaise de Sciences*, 23 vols. (The Hague, 1888–1950), 10:228, quoted in Maddison, *Life*, 191–92. "I will be astonished if Mr. Boyle, who has so many good experiments, will not be able to arrive at any theory of chemistry, after having meditated on it so much. However, in his books and as for all the conclusions which he draws from these observations, he has concluded only that which we know all to know—that all is accomplished mechanically. He is perhaps too reserved. Excellent men ought to leave us their conjectures, and it is wrong if they are not willing to impart anything but certain truths" (my translation). Note how Leibniz reread Boyle's attitude toward "certain knowledge."

50. Huygens to Leibniz, 4 February 1691/92, in *Oeuvres complètes de Christiaan Huygens*, 10:239. "Mr. Boyle is dead, as you will hear, no doubt. It appears so strange that he has constructed nothing upon so many of the experiments of which his books are full; but it is a difficult matter, and I have never believed that which he accomplished by establishing probabilistic principles capable of a very large practical application. He has, however, done well in contradicting those [principles] of the chemists" (my translation).

51. Clericuzio, "Redefinition," 581. Clericuzio suggests that Boyle felt mercury to be a likely candidate for designation as a primary substance, but he never stated this in other than very conjectural terms.

BIBLIOGRAPHY

Primary Sources

Manuscripts

The Royal Society of London

MS. 1. Oldenburg, Henry. Commonplace Book. 1660.

MSS. 194, 195, 199. Boyle, Robert. Commonplace books.

Boyle Letters (BL).

Boyle Papers (BP).

Printed Sources

Aristotle. *Generation of Animals.*

———. *Meteorologia.*

Birch, Thomas. *History of the Royal Society.* 4 vols. London, 1757.

Boerhaave, Hermann. *A New Method of Chemistry.* Translated by Peter Shaw and E. Chambers. London, 1727.

Boyle, Robert. *The Works of the Honorable Robert Boyle.* 1722. Edited by Thomas Birch. 6 vols. Hildesheim: Georg Olms, 1966.

Descartes, René. *Discourse on Method.* Translated by Laurence J. Lafleur. New York: Bobbs-Merrill, 1956.

———. *Principles of Philosophy.* Translated by Valentine Rodger Miller and Reese P. Miller. Dordrecht: Reidel, 1983

Diemerbroeck, Isbrand van. *A Treatise concerning the Pestilence.* Translated by Thomas Stanton. London, 1722.

[Greatraks, Valentine.] *A Brief Account of Mr. Valentine Greatraks, and Divers of the Strange Cases by Him Lately Performed.* London, 1666.

Hartlib, Samuel. *Chymical, Medicinal, and Chyrurgical Addresses made to S. Hartlib.* London, 1655.

Highmore, Nathaniel. *The History of Generation . . . To which is joyned a Discourse of the Cure of Wounds by Sympathy.* London, 1651.

Hoffmann, Friedrich. *Fundamenta Medicinae.* Translated with an introduction by Lester S. King. New York: Neale Watson, 1971.

Huygens, Christian. *Oeuvres complètes de Christiaan Huygens, publiées par la Société Hollandaise de Sciences.* 23 vols. The Hague, 1888–1950.

Lower, Richard. *Tractatus de corde item de motu et colore sanguinis et chyli in eum transitu.* London, 1669.

Pepys, Samuel. *The Diary of Samuel Pepys.* Edited by Robert Latham and William Matthews. 11 vols. London: G. Bell, 1970–83.

Pharmacopoeia Londinensis. London, 1618.

Plattes, Gabriel. *A Description of the Famous Kingdome of Macaria.* London, 1641.

Shaw, Peter. *An enquiry into the contents, virtues and uses of the Scarborough Spaw waters, with the method of examining any other mineral water.* London, 1734.

Starkey, George. *Pyrotechny Asserted and Illustrated.* London, 1658.

Sydenham, Thomas. *The Works of Thomas Sydenham, M.D.* Translated and edited by R. G. Latham. 2 vols. London: Sydenham Society, 1848–50.

Willis, Thomas. *Affectionum quae dicituntur hystericae et hypocondriacae . . . cui accesserunt exercitationes medico-physicae duae.* London, 1670.

Secondary Sources

Ackerknecht, Erwin H. *A Short History of Medicine.* Rev. ed. Baltimore: Johns Hopkins University Press, 1982.

Adelmann, Howard B. *Marcello Malpighi and the Evolution of Embryology.* 5 vols. Ithaca: Cornell University Press, 1966.

Bates, Donald G. "Thomas Willis and the Epidemic Fever of 1661: A Commentary." *Bulletin of the History of Medicine* 39 (1965): 393–414.

Benjamin, Marina. "Medicine, Morality, and the Politics of Berkeley's Tar-Water." In *Medical Enlightenment of the Eighteenth Century,* 165–93. *See* Cunningham, "Medicine to Calm the Mind."

Boas, Marie. *See* Hall, Marie Boas.

Boss, Jeffrey. "The 'Methodus Medendi' as an Index of Change in the Philosophy of Medical Science in the Sixteenth and Seventeenth Centuries." *History and Philosophy of the Life Sciences* 1 (1979): 13–42.

Bullough, Vern L. *The Development of Medicine as a Profession.* New York: S. Karger, 1966.

Canny, Nicholas. *The Upstart Earl: A Study of the Social and Mental World of Richard Boyle, First Earl of Cork: 1566–1643.* Cambridge: Cambridge University Press, 1982.

Carter, Richard B. *Descartes' Medical Philosophy: The Organic Solution to the Mind-Body Problem.* Baltimore: Johns Hopkins University Press, 1983.

Cassedy, James H. "Medicine and the Rise of Statistics." In *Medicine in Seventeenth Century England,* 283–312. *See* Debus, "Paracelsian Medicine."

Chalmers, Gordon K. "Effluvia, the History of a Metaphor." *Modern Language Association of America Publications* 52 (1937): 1031–50.

———. "The Lodestone and the Understanding of Matter in Seventeenth Century England." *Philosophy of Science* 4 (1937): 75–95.

———. "Three Terms of the Corpuscularian Philosophy." *Modern Philology* 33 (1936): 243–60.

Clericuzio, Antonio. "A Redefinition of Boyle's Chemistry and Corpuscular Philosophy." *Annals of Science* 47 (1990): 561–89.

Coley, Noel G. "Physicians and the Chemical Analysis of Mineral Waters in Eighteenth-Century England." *Medical History* 26 (1982): 123–44.

Cook, Harold J. *Decline of the Old Medical Regime in Stuart London.* Ithaca: Cornell University Press, 1986.

———. "Physicians and the New Philosophy: Henry Stubbe and the Virtuosi-Physicians." In *The Medical Revolution of the Seventeenth Century,* edited by Roger French and Andrew Wear, 246–71. Cambridge: Cambridge University Press, 1989.

Crombie, A. C. *Medieval and Early Modern Science.* 2 vols. Garden City, N.Y.: Doubleday Anchor Books, 1959.

Cunningham, Andrew. "Medicine to Calm the Mind: Boerhaave's Medical System, and Why It Was Adopted in Edinburgh." In *The Medical Enlightenment of the Eighteenth Century,* edited by Andrew Cunningham and Roger French, 40–66. Cambridge: Cambridge University Press, 1990.

———. "Thomas Sydenham: Epidemics, Experiment, and the 'Good Old Cause.'" In *Medical Revolution of the Seventeenth Century,* 164–90. *See* Cook, "Physicians and the New Philosophy."

Debus, Allen G. *The Chemical Philosophy: Paracelsian Science and Medicine in the Sixteenth and Seventeenth Centuries.* 2 vols. New York: Science History Publications, 1977.

———. *The English Paracelsians.* New York: Neale Watson, 1965.

———. "Paracelsian Medicine: Noah Biggs and the Problem of Medical Reform." In *Medicine in Seventeenth Century England: A Symposium held at UCLA in Honor of C. D. O'Malley,* edited by Allen Debus, 34–38. Berkeley and Los Angeles: University of California Press, 1974.

Dewhurst, Kenneth. *Dr. Thomas Sydenham (1624–1689): His Life and Writings.* Berkeley: University of California Press, 1966.

Dobbs, Betty Jo. "Studies in the Natural Philosophy of Sir Kenelm Digby. Part I." *Ambix* 18 (1971): 1–25.

Elmer, Peter. "Medicine, Religion, and the Puritan Revolution." In *Medical Revolution of the Seventeenth Century,* 10–45. *See* Cook, "Physicians and the New Philosophy."

Fisch, H. "The Scientist as Priest: A Note on Robert Boyle's Natural Theology." *Isis* 15 (1953): 252–65.

Frank, Robert G. *Harvey and the Oxford Physiologists: A Study of Scientific Ideas.* Berkeley and Los Angeles: University of California Press, 1980.

———. "John Aubrey, F.R.S., John Lydall, and Science at Commonwealth Oxford." *Notes and Records of the Royal Society of London* 27 (1973): 193–217.

French, Roger. "Sickness and the Soul: Stahl, Hoffmann, and Sauvages on Pathology." In *Medical Enlightenment of the Eighteenth Century,* 88–137. *See* Cunningham, "Medicine to Calm the Mind."

Fulton, John F. *A Bibliography of the Honorable Robert Boyle.* 2d ed. Oxford: Clarendon Press, 1961.

Gascoigne, John. "A Reappraisal of the Role of the Universities in the Scientific Revolution." In *Reappraisals of the Scientific Revolution,* edited by David C. Lindberg and Robert S. Westman, 207–60. Cambridge: Cambridge University Press, 1990.

Gelbart, Nina Rattner. "The Intellectual Development of Walter Charleton." *Ambix* 18 (1971): 149–68.

Gieryn, Thomas. "Distancing Science from Religion in Seventeenth-Century England." *Isis* 79 (1988): 582–93.

Glacken, Clarence J. *Traces on the Rhodian Shore: Nature and Culture in Western Thought from Ancient Times to the End of the Eighteenth Century.* Berkeley and Los Angeles: University of California Press, 1973.

Guerlac, Henry. "John Mayow and the Aerial Niter: Studies in the Chemistry of John Mayow, I." *Actes du Septième Congrès International d'Histoire des Sciences.* Jerusalem, 1953. Pp. 332–39.

———. "Studies in the Chemistry of John Mayow: II. The Poet's Nitre." *Isis* 45 (1954): 243–55.

Guerrini, Anita. "Isaac Newton, George Cheyne, and the *Principia Medicinae.*" In *Medical Revolution of the Seventeenth Century,* 222–45. *See* Cook, "Physicians and the New Philosophy."

———. "Newtonian Matter Theory, Chemistry, and Medicine, 1690–1713." Ph.D. diss., Indiana University, 1983.

Hall, A. Rupert. "Medicine and the Royal Society." In *Medicine in Seventeenth Century England,* 421–52. *See* Debus, "Paracelsian Medicine."

Hall, Marie Boas. "Boyle's Method of Work: Promoting His Corpuscular Philosophy." *Notes and Records of the Royal Society of London* 41 (1987): 111–43.

———. "An Early Version of Boyle's Sceptical Chymist." *Isis* 45 (1954): 153–68.

———. "The Establishment of the Mechanical Philosophy." *Osiris* 10 (1952): 412–541.

———. *Robert Boyle and Seventeenth-Century Chemistry.* Cambridge: Cambridge University Press, 1958.

Hall, Thomas S. *Ideas of Life and Matter: Studies in the History of General Physiology, 600 B.C.–1900 A.D.* 2 vols. Chicago: University of Chicago Press, 1969.

Harwood, John T., ed. *The Early Essays and Ethics of Robert Boyle.* Carbondale: Southern Illinois University Press, 1991.

Henry, John. "Occult Qualities and the Experimental Philosophy: Active Principles in Pre-Newtonian Matter Theory." *History of Science* 24 (1986): 335–81.

Holmes, Frederic L. *Claude Bernard and Animal Chemistry: The Emergence of a Scientist.* Cambridge: Harvard University Press, 1974.

Hunter, Michael. "Alchemy, Magic, and Moralism in the Thought of Robert Boyle." *British Journal for the History of Science* 23 (1990): 387–410.

———. *The Royal Society and Its Fellows, 1660–1700: The Morphology of an Early Scientific Institution.* British Society for the History of Science Monograph, 4. London, 1982.

———. *Science and Society in Restoration England.* Cambridge: Cambridge University Press, 1981.

Jacob, James R. *Robert Boyle and the English Revolution: A Study in Social and Intellectual Change.* New York: Burt Franklin, 1977.

Jacob, James R., and Margaret C. Jacob. "The Anglican Origins of Modern Science: The Metaphysical Foundations of the Whig Constitution." *Isis* 71 (1980): 251–67.

Jewson, N. D. "The Disappearance of the Sick Man from Medical Cosmology, 1770–1870." *Sociology* 10 (1976): 225–40.

———. "Medical Knowledge and the Patronage System in Eighteenth-Century England." *Sociology* 8 (1974): 369–85.

Kaplan, Barbara Beigun. "Greatrakes the Stroker: The Interpretations of His Contemporaries." *Isis* 73 (1982): 178–85.

Kargon, Robert. *Atomism in England from Hariot to Newton.* Oxford: Clarendon Press, 1966.

Keele, Kenneth D. "The Sydenham-Boyle Theory of Morbific Particles." *Medical History* 18 (1974): 240–48.

King, Lester. *The Growth of Medical Thought.* Chicago: University of Chicago Press, 1963.

———. *The Road to Medical Enlightenment.* New York: Science History Publications, 1970.

McKie, Douglas. "Fire and the Flamma Vitalis: Boyle, Hooke, and Mayow." In *Science, Medicine, and History: Essays in Honour of Charles Singer,* edited by E. A. Underwood. 2 vols. London: Oxford University Press, 1953.

———. "The Origins and Foundation of the Royal Society of London." *Notes and Records of the Royal Society of London* 15 (1960): 1–37.

Maddison, R. E. W. *The Life of the Honourable Robert Boyle.* New York: Barnes & Noble, 1969.

Mandelbaum, Maurice. *Philosophy, Science, and Sense Perception: Historical and Critical Studies.* Baltimore: Johns Hopkins Press, 1964.

Meinel, Christoph. "Empirical Support for the Corpuscular Theory in the Seventeenth Century." In *Theory and Experiment: Recent Insights and New Perspectives on Their Relation,* edited by Diderik Batens and Jean Paul van Bendegem, 77–92. Dordrecht: Reidel, 1988.

Merchant, Carolyn. *The Death of Nature: Women, Ecology, and the Scientific Revolution.* New York: Harper & Row, 1980.

Merton, Thomas K. *Science, Technology, and Society in Seventeenth Century England.* New York: Harper & Row, 1970.

More, Louis Trenchard. *The Life and Works of the Honourable Robert Boyle.* London: Oxford University Press, 1944.

Mulligan, Lotte. "'Reason,' 'Right Reason,' and 'Revelation' in Mid-Seventeenth Century England." In *Occult and Scientific Mentalities in the Renaissance,* edited by Brian Vickers, 375–401. Cambridge: Cambridge University Press, 1984.

Mulligan, Lotte, and Glenn Mulligan. "Reconstructing Restoration Science." *Social Studies of Science* 11 (1981): 327–64.

Nicolson, Malcolm. "The Metastatic Theory of Pathogenesis and the Professional Interests of the Eighteenth-Century Physician." *Medical History* 32 (1988): 277–300.

Niebyl, Peter. "Sennert, Van Helmont, and Medical Ontology." *Bulletin of the History of Medicine* 45 (1971): 115–37.

O'Brien, John J. "Samuel Hartlib's Influence on Robert Boyle's Scientific Development. Part I: The Stalbridge Period." *Annals of Science* 21 (1965): 1–14.

Oster, Malcolm R. "The 'Beaume of Diuinity': Animal Suffering in the Early Thought of Robert Boyle." *British Journal for the History of Science* 22 (1989): 151–79.

Partington, J. R. *A Short History of Chemistry.* 3d ed. New York: Harper Torchbooks, 1960.

Porter, Dorothy, and Roy Porter. *Patients' Progress: Doctors and Doctoring in Eighteenth Century England.* Stanford, Calif.: Stanford University Press, 1989.

Porter, Roy. "The Early Royal Society and the Spread of Medical Knowledge." In *Medical Revolution of the Seventeenth Century,* 272–93. *See* Cook, "Physicians and the New Philosophy."

———. "Lay Medical Knowledge in the Eighteenth Century: The Evidence of *The Gentlemen's Magazine.*" *Medical History* 29 (1958): 138–68.

Purver, Margery. *The Royal Society: Concept and Creation.* Cambridge: MIT Press, 1967.

Riley, James C. *The Eighteenth Century Campaign to Avoid Disease.* New York: Macmillan, 1987.

Romanell, Patrick. *John Locke and Medicine: A New Key to Locke.* Buffalo, N.Y.: Prometheus Books, 1984.

Rowbottom, Margaret E. "The Earliest Published Writing of Robert Boyle." *Annals of Science* 6 (1948–50): 376–89.

Sargent, Frederick. *Hippocratic Heritage: A History of Ideas about Weather and Human Health.* New York: Pergamon, 1982.

Schaffer, Simon. "Measuring Virtue: Eudiometry, Enlightenment, and Pneumatic Medicine." In *Medical Enlightenment of the Eighteenth Century,* 281–318. *See* Cunningham, "Medicine to Calm the Mind."

Shapere, Dudley. "Plausibility and Justification in the Development of Science." *Journal of Philosophy* 63 (1966): 611–27.

Shapin, Steven. "The House of Experiment in Seventeenth-Century England." *Isis* 79 (1988): 373–404.

———. "Social Uses of Science." In *The Ferment of Knowledge: Studies in the Historiography of Eighteenth Century Science,* edited by G. S. Rousseau and Roy Porter, 93–139. Cambridge: Cambridge University Press, 1980.

———. "Understanding the Merton Thesis." *Isis* 79 (1988): 594–605.

Shapin, Steven, and Simon Schaffer. *Leviathan and the Air-Pump: Hobbes, Boyle, and the Experimental Life.* Princeton: Princeton University Press, 1985.

Shapiro, Barbara J. "Latitudinarianism and Science in Seventeenth Century England." In Webster, *Intellectual Revolution of the Seventeenth Century,* 286–316.

Stimson, Dorothy. *Scientists and Amateurs: A History of the Royal Society.* New York: Henry Schuman, 1948.

Syfret, R. H. "The Origins of the Royal Society." *Notes and Records of the Royal Society of London* 5 (1948): 75–137.

Temkin, Owsei. "The Scientific Approach to Disease: Specific Entities and Individual Sickness." In *The Double Face of Janus,* 441–55. Baltimore: Johns Hopkins University Press, 1977.

Trevor-Roper, H. R. "Three Foreigners and the Philosophy of the English Revolution." *Encounter* 14 (1960): 3–20.

Turnbull, G. H. *Hartlib, Dury, and Comenius: Gleanings from Hartlib's Papers.* Liverpool: Liverpool University Press, 1947.

———. "Samuel Hartlib's Influence on the Early History of the Royal Society." *Notes and Records of the Royal Society of London* 10 (1953): 101–30.

Van Leeuwen, Henry G. *The Problem of Certainty in English Thought, 1630–1690.* The Hague: Martinus Nijhoff, 1963.

Van Melsen, Andrew G. *From Atomos to Atom.* New York: Harper Torchbooks, 1960.

Webster, Charles. "English Medical Reformers of the Puritan Revolution." *Ambix* 14 (1967): 16–41.

———. *The Great Instauration: Science, Medicine, and Reform, 1626–1660.* New York: Holmes & Meier, 1975.

———. "New Light on the Invisible College: The Social Relations of English Science in the Mid-Seventeenth Century." *Transactions of the Royal Historical Society* 24 (1974): 19–42.

———. *Samuel Hartlib and the Advancement of Learning.* Cambridge: Cambridge University Press, 1970.

Webster, Charles, ed. *The Intellectual Revolution of the Seventeenth Century.* London: Routledge & Kegan Paul, 1974.

Westfall, Richard S. "Newton and the Hermetic Tradition." In *Science, Medicine, and Society in the Renaissance: Essays to Honour Walter Pagel,* edited by Allen G. Debus, 2:183–88. 2 vols. New York: Science History Publications, 1972.

———. *Science and Religion in Seventeenth-Century England.* Ann Arbor: University of Michigan Press, 1973.

———. "Unpublished Boyle Papers Relating to Scientific Method." *Annals of Science* 12 (1956): 63–73, 103–17.

Wolfe, David E. "Sydenham and Locke on the Limits of Anatomy." *Bulletin of the History of Medicine* 35 (1961): 193–220.

Yates, Frances A. *The Rosicrucian Enlightenment.* London: Routledge & Kegan Paul, 1972.

INDEX

Index

Index